MW00585959

Clinical Chemistry

Quality in Laboratory Diagnosis

Diagnostic Standards of Care

MICHAEL LAPOSATA, MD, PHD
Series Editor

Coagulation Disorders
Quality in Laboratory Diagnosis
Michael Laposata, MD, PhD

Clinical Microbiology
Quality in Laboratory Diagnosis
Charles W. Stratton, MD

Laboratory Management
Quality in Laboratory Diagnosis
Candis A. Kinkus

Transfusion Medicine
Quality in Laboratory Diagnosis
Quentin G. Eichbaum, MD, PhD, MPH, MFA, FCAP
Garrett S. Booth, MD, MS
Pampee P. Young, MD, PhD

Clinical Chemistry
Quality in Laboratory Diagnosis
James H. Nichols, PhD, DABCC, FACB
Carol A. Rauch, MD, PhD, FCAP

Forthcoming in the Series
Hematology/Immunology

Diagnostic Standards of Care Series

Clinical Chemistry
Quality in Laboratory Diagnosis

James H. Nichols, PhD, DABCC, FACB
Professor of Pathology, Microbiology, and Immunology
Medical Director of Clinical Chemistry
Vanderbilt University School of Medicine
Nashville, Tennessee

Carol A. Rauch, MD, PhD, FCAP
Associate Professor of Pathology, Microbiology, and Immunology
Associate Medical Director of Clinical Laboratories
Associate Medical Director of Vanderbilt Pathology Laboratory
  Services
Vanderbilt University School of Medicine
Nashville, Tennessee

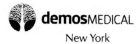 **demos**MEDICAL
New York

Visit our website at www.demosmedpub.com

ISBN: 978-1-62070-030-3
e-book ISBN: 978-1-61705-189-0

Acquisitions Editor: Richard Winters
Compositor: S4Carlisle Publishing Services

Medicine is an ever-changing science. Research and clinical experience are continually expanding our knowledge, in particular our understanding of proper treatment and drug therapy. The authors, editors, and publisher have made every effort to ensure that all information in this book is in accordance with the state of knowledge at the time of production of the book. Nevertheless, the authors, editors, and publisher are not responsible for errors or omissions or for any consequences from application of the information in this book and make no warranty, expressed or implied, with respect to the contents of the publication. Every reader should examine carefully the package inserts accompanying each drug and should carefully check whether the dosage schedules mentioned therein or the contraindications stated by the manufacturer differ from the statements made in this book. Such examination is particularly important with drugs that are either rarely used or have been newly released on the market.

Library of Congress Cataloging-in-Publication Data

Nichols, James H., 1961– author.
  Clinical chemistry : quality in laboratory diagnosis / James H. Nichols, Carol A. Rauch.
     p. ; cm. — (Diagnostic standards of care)
  Includes bibliographical references and index.
  ISBN 978-1-62070-030-3—ISBN 1-62070-030-1—ISBN 978-1-61705-189-0 (e-book)
  I. Rauch, Carol A., author. II. Title. III. Series: Diagnostic standards of care.
  [DNLM: 1. Chemistry, Clinical. 2. Clinical Chemistry Tests—methods. QY 90]
  RB40
  616.07'56—dc23
                                        2013021660

Printed in the United States of America by Bradford & Bigelow.
13 14 15 16 17 / 5 4 3 2 1

Contents

Series Foreword

"Above all, do no harm." This frequently quoted admonition to health care providers is highly regarded, but despite that, there are few books, if any, that focus primarily on how to avoid harming patients by learning from the mistakes of others.

Would it not be of great benefit to patients if all health care providers were aware of the thrombotic consequences from heparin-induced thrombocytopenia before a patient's leg is amputated? The clinically significant, often lethal, thrombotic events that occur in patients who develop heparin-induced thrombocytopenia would be greatly diminished if all health care providers appropriately monitored platelet counts in patients being treated with intravenous unfractionated heparin.

It was a desire to learn from the mistakes of others that led to the concept for this series of books on diagnostic standards of care. As the test menu in the clinical laboratory has enlarged in size and complexity, errors in selection of tests and errors in the interpretation of test results have become commonplace, and these mistakes can result in poor patient outcomes. This series of books on diagnostic standards of care in coagulation, microbiology, transfusion medicine, hematology, clinical chemistry, immunology, and laboratory management are all organized in a similar fashion. Clinical errors, and accompanying cases to illustrate each error, are presented within all of the chapters in several discrete categories: errors in test selection, errors in result interpretation, other errors, and diagnostic controversies. Each chapter concludes with a summary list of the standards of care. The most common errors made by thousands of health care providers daily are the ones that have been selected for presentation in this series of books.

Practicing physicians ordering tests with which they are less familiar would benefit significantly by learning of the potential errors associated with ordering such tests and errors associated with interpreting an infrequently encountered test result. Medical trainees who are gaining clinical experience would benefit significantly by first understanding what not to do when it comes to ordering laboratory tests and interpreting test results from the clinical laboratory. Individuals working in the clinical laboratory would also benefit by learning of the common mistakes made by health care providers so that they are better able to provide helpful advice that would avert the damaging consequences of an error. Finally, laboratory managers and hospital administrators would benefit by having knowledge of test ordering mistakes to improve the efficiency of the clinical laboratory and avoid the cost of performing unnecessary tests.

If the errors described in this series of books could be greatly reduced, the savings to the health care system and the improvement in patient outcomes would be dramatic.

Michael Laposata, MD, PhD
Series Editor

Preface

Why do errors occur in the laboratory and how do we detect and prevent erroneous results from affecting patient care? In the complex setting of the modern laboratory, errors can occur in the preanalytical, analytical, and postanalytical phases of the testing process. Good laboratory practice now dictates much of our laboratory policies and procedures. New instrumentation incorporates the latest methodologies to prevent errors within the laboratory setting. Automated analyzers utilize specimen barcoding to order tests, aliquot samples, perform analyses, and report results, totally without human intervention. However, if the specimen is labeled with another patient's identification, all of the analytical error prevention systems will not prevent the right result from being reported to the wrong patient. If and when this occurs, there is potential for a variety of adverse events for the patient. Thus, laboratory policies must expand beyond the walls of the physical laboratory to incorporate preanalytical and postanalytical processes, involving other departments and partners in delivery of health care. Good laboratory practice must become an integral part of good "hospital" or "clinic" practice and incorporate interdisciplinary collaboration in the effort to reduce error. Many of our laboratory processes are dependent on the quality practices of staff outside of the laboratory. Proper patient identification and appropriate specimen labeling by nursing and phlebotomy staff on the unit are critical to the error-prevention mechanisms incorporated into modern, automated laboratory systems. We can therefore not work alone! We are dependent, now more than ever, on our clinical colleagues to prevent medical errors related to laboratory testing. Truly effective, good laboratory practice requires a total quality management systems approach. Without all departments working in concert, errors will continue to occur.

How do we incorporate good laboratory practice into our systems? First, we must educate our clinical colleagues about our experiences and insight. Laboratory technologists, managers, and directors uniquely understand sources of error, as knowledge and insight are gained by experience and informed by understanding of laboratory processes. On the other hand, clinicians are keenly attuned to the need for laboratory tests to support the diagnosis and continuing care of a patient. We must find a common ground to communicate our mutual knowledge and experience for the benefit of the patient. Broadly speaking, we need to define good laboratory practices across the health system. Regardless of where or how a test is conducted, fundamental principles of patient safety should apply to prevent all sources of error. Finally, we must learn from our mistakes in order to advance to a higher level of quality. Trends should not go unnoticed, and corrective actions should be mandated for errors to prevent their recurrence in the care of other patients.

This book illustrates cases where the system broke down. For whatever reason, personnel were not diligent, policies were not in place, or quality was not sufficiently monitored. In each case the system failed, and we should learn from these experiences. Patients may have been harmed, people may have been blamed, but the system surrounding them was not meeting their needs. Errors are and will continue to be inherent in all human processes; we need to create systems that detect and prevent errors from reaching the patient. This book is intended to highlight how systems can fail, so that broader organizations that include the laboratory can be proactive in developing robust mechanisms to prevent error.

James H. Nichols, PhD, DABCC, FACB
Carol A. Rauch, MD, PhD, FCAP

Acknowledgments

The authors wish to acknowledge the technologists and management staff in the clinical laboratories for identifying these cases and for their support and dedication to quality patient care. The cases reported in this book are real, although names have been changed, and identification of these issues led to performance improvement. It is our hope that by sharing these experiences, we can increase awareness of potential weaknesses and further quality improvement efforts in other laboratories. We sincerely appreciate the guidance received from our series editor, Dr. Michael Laposata.

1 Specimen Receiving and Processing

OVERVIEW

The specimen receiving and processing area of the laboratory is the entry point for specimens into the laboratory. As the initial contact point, processing staff may examine a specimen and detect common preanalytical errors before the specimen is analyzed. Mislabeling, wrong tube types, transportation delays, and other mistakes can affect patient results. By detecting and correcting problems before the specimen is placed on an analyzer, staff can prevent clinical mismanagement based on erroneous results. Receiving a quality specimen is the first step toward ensuring a quality result.

PREANALYTICAL ERRORS

Labeling Errors

▶ A large clinical laboratory receives thousands of specimens each day. Specimens can look alike, because blood in a common collection tube does not look different from another sample of blood in the same type of tube. The specimen label is the only means of distinguishing among specimens. Clinicians may envision their patient as the only one being analyzed by the laboratory, but in today's highly automated clinical laboratory, specimens are lined up and analyzed solely based on the label/barcode on the side of the tube. Often, an operator must retrieve individual specimens if they are needed for reanalysis or additional testing. Searching for a specific specimen among racks of similar specimens can be labor intensive, so automated processes that archive and manage specimen storage and retrieval can improve the laboratory's efficiency. These additional processes are also based on information contained on the specimen label. Thus, clinicians must ensure that patients are properly identified and specimens are uniquely and appropriately labeled before sending them to the laboratory. Otherwise, specimen mix-ups may occur and can lead to reporting erroneous results, and in turn to adverse events for the patient.

Case with Error

A blood gas specimen is received in the laboratory with no label. The syringe was tightly capped and sent to the laboratory through the hospital pneumatic tube system. Several specimens arrived from the same nursing unit in the pneumatic tube at the same time, each patient's specimen arriving in an individual biohazard transport bag. The specimen in question arrived in a single, patient-specific transport bag with a completed requisition, but no label on the syringe. The physician was called, and she requested that the lab just label the tube so the test could be run. Sample collection from this patient posed a challenge for the phlebotomist, and the patient had to be stuck twice to obtain this specimen. The laboratory explained the hospital policy against relabeling specimens, but offered to analyze the specimen under the condition that a comment noting the specimen labeling error be appended to the results for the benefit of those who might utilize the result in the future. The physician was a resident and did not want his attending to see the error comment, so the specimen was canceled and re-collected.

The next sample on this patient arrived in the laboratory about an hour later. This specimen was labeled, but arrived without a test requisition. In addition, transport to the laboratory was delayed more than 45 minutes after collection. Blood gas specimens must be transported to the laboratory immediately after collection (within 30 minutes), unless the specimen is transported on ice. This specimen arrived at room temperature through the pneumatic tube. The laboratory called the physician again to cancel this specimen. The physician became irate and threatened the laboratory manager, who handed the phone over to the laboratory director. The laboratory director explained the policy and sympathized with the physician over the difficulty of obtaining specimens from this patient. The laboratory offered to analyze the specimen for electrolytes, glucose, and creatinine, but indicated that the blood gases, pH, and ionized calcium would not be valid after such a delay. Since the physician required blood gases for clinical management, the patient had to be stuck a fourth time. This time, the physician had a nurse walk the specimen to the laboratory to ensure specimen acceptability.

Explanation and Consequences

Physicians may get upset with the laboratory and may perceive laboratory policies that are intended to support patient safety as obstructive. Although the laboratory sometimes refuses a physician's request, institutions have policies and procedures to ensure reliable results. These policies contribute to patient safety by preventing the analysis of compromised specimens that could lead to incorrect and misleading test results, and subsequent inappropriate medical actions.

Unlabeled specimens can originate from any patient. There is little guarantee that an unlabeled specimen actually belongs to a "suspected" patient, particularly with the volume of patients that are seen in busy physician offices, hospitals, and health care facilities. Physicians may request the laboratory to relabel and analyze an unlabeled or mislabeled specimen, but correcting the label does not resolve the fundamental uncertainty of patient identity. Changing the specimen label actually complicates the labeling issue by altering the actual specimen that arrived in the laboratory. A better option is to preserve the specimen label as it was received. This provides documentation of how the specimen arrived to the laboratory and supports any labeling questions raised. Discussion of a specimen identity issue with the ordering physician may help determine the best resolution of the problem, and such conversations need involvement by someone in the laboratory with sufficient authority and responsibility to make individualized decisions about specimen processing. Many times, a specimen may be ordered, collected, and labeled by staff under another person's authority. Nurses may order tests for physicians, or students may order for the attending on the unit. Discussions with the physicians of record are necessary to alert them to a labeling error and help determine the best course of action for the specimen.

When specimens are found to be acceptable for analysis, any specimen identification uncertainties should be noted as a comment with the test result. Labeling comments are important alerts because they warn of the potential for errors in specimen labeling to those interpreting the results. In a physician's office, because a limited number of staff may have access to view results, labeling issues with individual samples may be more easily communicated and resolved in this setting. However, for hospitalized patients, since multiple physicians, residents, and staff may be involved in a patient's care and have access to test results, they all must know that a patient identification may be suspect.

> ▶ Labeling errors can encompass a variety of mistakes beyond unlabeled specimens. Samples can be mislabeled with another patient's name or contain incorrect information, such as name misspelling or wrong demographics such as age or sex. Partially labeled specimens contain two appropriate

identifiers, but may be missing important information, such as specimen source or date/time of collection. Illegible labels that have been smudged or partially destroyed are also commonly encountered. Institutions should have a specimen labeling policy to determine how labeling errors will be handled. Some cases may present unique situations that require individual consideration, despite the existence of a labeling policy.

Case with Error

The laboratory receives a call from an outpatient orthopedics clinic that the test results reported for a patient may not belong to that patient. Fluid analysis and microbiology results on a joint aspirate of the left knee for John Smith actually belong to Rebecca Johnson. Both patients were seen in the clinic yesterday with knee complaints, but only Rebecca Johnson had joint fluid collected. John Smith was discharged without a procedure. The clinic requests that the test results be moved from John Smith's medical record to Rebecca Johnson's record. This is the second specimen mislabeling to occur in the last 2 weeks from this clinic.

Explanation and Consequences

Laboratories should carefully consider how they handle mislabeled test results. A joint fluid is an unusual sample that cannot easily be re-collected. If the mislabeling is noted before analysis, the test could be analyzed and the test result commented in order to alert staff to the labeling issue. However, when the identity of a test result comes into question after analysis, the laboratory should never move the test from one patient's medical record to another patient's chart. That result has been released and visible to clinicians for some period of time on a specific patient's record. Removing the result entirely from a patient's record could create a conflict if treatment or other care decisions have already been made based on the result. A good practice would indicate that a specific result was reported incorrectly at a particular date/time and actually belonged to another patient. Such a comment would immediately alert clinicians of the labeling error. This would prevent clinicians from taking further action without completely removing the test from the patient's record. By replacing the test result with a comment, staff would be warned of the error and also preserve the original report should a question about the result arise in the future.

The test result should also not be moved to another patient's medical record, because the identity of the test result is now in question. While the result may not belong to John Smith, there is no evidence that it actually belongs to Rebecca Johnson. The laboratory has only the specimen label in writing under John Smith's name, and a verbal conversation with clinic staff to support the true specimen identity. While some hospitals may request completion of an error report prior to moving a result, best practice would result in the test only as a comment in Rebecca's record (without the actual test result), indicating the mislabeling communication that took place with the name of the clinic staff and date/time of the call, and include reference to the specimen identification number that could trace the result to the other patient's record. In this manner, the result trail is preserved from the label on the specimen received in the laboratory through analysis and reporting of the result, as well as correction of the result after reporting in the medical record of both patients within the electronic record.

Since this clinic had multiple occurrences of specimen mislabeling, the laboratory should offer continuing education to avoid additional problems in the future. Physicians routinely collect the specimens, set the unlabeled containers on a shelf outside the examination room, and support staff later label the specimens and complete the test requisitions on behalf of the physician when there is time down the hall at a work station. This process could easily lead to mislabeling opportunities when exam rooms turn over with new patients before the specimens are labeled. The key to quality specimen results is maintaining the integrity of specimen identification from patient through collection, analysis, and reporting of results. The person collecting the specimen should identify the patient using a minimum of two different identifiers such as full name and date of birth or medical record number. The specimen should then be labeled with the same unique identifiers in the presence of the patient at the bedside, immediately after collection. Passing the specimen to others for labeling presents an opportunity for error. Unlabeled specimens should never be stored in a common area like a hallway or a counter where there is a potential for mix-up with other specimens or labels.

> Specimen labeling errors may not be immediately apparent. Errors with one specimen may implicate that specimen in a labeling error and bring errors for multiple specimens into question. Thus, processing staff need to be diligent of the potential for mistakes and verify the integrity of specimen identification with each and every specimen arriving in the laboratory.

Case with Error

Two presurgical urine pregnancy tests arrive from an affiliate hospital on pediatric patients, Frances Smith, age 13, and Jennifer Richards, age 15. One of the urine specimens was light straw color and had two labels on opposite sides of the container, one for Frances Smith and the other for Jennifer Richards. The second specimen arriving in the courier delivery was a dark brown color and had the name Jennifer Richards on the sample. Since the identity of both specimens is now in question, the preoperative unit at the affiliate hospital was contacted with a request to re-collect both specimens. Staff indicated that they were holding surgery and anesthesia until the results of the pregnancy tests were available and requested that the laboratory rush the test performance.

The next two samples arrived by stat courier. One of the specimens was a light, straw color while the other specimen was dark brown. This time, both specimens contained a label for the same patient, Frances Smith. Given the previous specimens and the different color of the two current specimens, the preoperative unit was contacted again. The laboratory spoke with the nurse manager, explained the problem with the previous specimens, and the appearance of the current specimens. Staff would collect another set of specimens, and the nurse manager of the unit would observe the labeling.

The next set of samples arrived shortly. The straw-colored sample was labeled with Jennifer Richards' name and the dark-colored urine was labeled Frances Smith. One of the patients was positive for pregnancy creating a greater concern for everyone involved, given the previous specimen mix-ups and the age of the patients. Both results were verified under the name of the final set of samples. All previous test requests were canceled with a comment noting possible mislabeling and need for specimen re-collection. The case was sent to the affiliate hospital's quality management office for follow-up.

Explanation and Consequences

On review of the case, staffing on the day of surgery was expected to be short due to planned vacations. Workers from the previous night attempted to streamline patient admissions the following morning by prelabeling the collection containers and completing the requisitions in advance, trying to be helpful to the morning operations. Yet, despite the good intentions, in the rush to prepare patients for surgery in the morning, they did not notice that extra labels had already been printed and the specimen containers were already labeled. The morning staff simply followed their routine practice, identified patients, printed labels, and labeled the specimens as they always would. Staff did not expect the specimen containers to already be labeled and did not check to verify the labels already on the containers. In the morning, operations were very delayed and in the rush to expedite the surgeries, the operating room staff failed again to double-check their labeling.

This case exemplifies the need for a labeling process that is explicitly followed each time a specimen is collected so that each specimen is already linked to the correct patient and results can be safely entered into the patient's records. Shortcuts, like prelabeling tubes, present the opportunity for error and must be avoided. Specimens should be labeled in the presence of a patient to ensure the specimen label matches the positive patient identification. Once a urine specimen is collected, staff should double-check that the identification on the specimen matches the patient prior to sending the specimen to the laboratory. Urine specimens should also be labeled on the side of the container and not on the lid, which could be separated from the sample, or exchanged or mixed with another lid in the laboratory during processing and analysis.

Collection in the Incorrect Tube Additive

> Specimen collection tubes are color coded to indicate different additives. Some additives prevent clotting and allow the analysis of plasma, while other additives inhibit glycolysis and metabolism. Color-coded tubes may also contain a gel barrier that facilitates sample processing. These different collection tubes have different intended purposes and are generally not interchangeable. Certain tests may require specific types of collection tubes, processing, or transport prior to analysis. Failure to follow the recommended collection and processing instructions can compromise the quality of test results.

Case with Error

A purple-top microtainer tube (0.5 mL volume) containing EDTA preservative arrives in the laboratory, but the requirements for the test requested specify collection in a red-top gel tube with no additives. The neonatal unit is contacted. Staff involved in specimen collection request the specimen be sent back to the unit. To comply, the laboratory processor sends the tube back to the unit after canceling the tests. The next specimen from the patient arrives about an hour later in the same purple-top EDTA microtainer, but this smaller tube was now pushed into a larger 10 mL red-top gel tube. The specimen is accompanied by a Patient Safety Report claiming possible patient harm; the allegation is that the laboratory delayed patient care by not running the tests requested and required more blood to be drawn from a neonatal patient.

Explanation and Consequences

The colored caps on specimen collection tubes indicate the type of specimen additive or preservative contained within the tube. The color coding is not simply a convenience that directs a tube to a specific section of the laboratory. Staff conducting phlebotomy should be familiar with the different types of collection tubes and test requirements. Sometimes phlebotomy staff is supervised by nursing administration ("decentralized" phlebotomy), and in other institutions phlebotomy is supervised by the laboratory ("centralized" phlebotomy). Under either organizational scheme, the laboratory should be directly involved to educate any staff performing phlebotomy so that they understand test requirements and preanalytical variation that can occur during specimen collection. Placing one tube inside another tube does not remove the EDTA additive in the blood sample. A new sample collected in the right type of tube is required for the specific tests requested. The laboratory is not obstructing patient care, but rather facilitating test result quality by refusing to analyze this specimen, since the EDTA in the wrong collection tube will prevent the true result for the patient from being generated.

Errors in Specimen Transportation

Delays in transportation or exposure of specimens to extreme temperatures during transit to a laboratory can affect test results. Laboratories need to provide recommendations for limiting the exposure of specimens to extreme temperatures prior to processing and analysis. Couriers should monitor environmental conditions to ensure that specimens are maintained within specified conditions. The quality of test results can be affected by preanalytical conditions.

Case with Error

A reference laboratory picks up specimens from a number of physician offices and health care settings within the region around the laboratory.

Since some of the clinics work different shifts, the reference laboratory provides drop boxes for specimen pickup after hours. These drop boxes are a simple metal box attached to the side of the building facing the parking lot to allow easy access to couriers driving between locations. Physician offices are encouraged to process and aliquot their specimens prior to pickup by the reference laboratory. Most of the offices use gel separator tubes, and simply centrifuge the specimens prior to dropping them in the box for pickup. The drop boxes are intended for use after hours, as couriers can pick up specimens within the office during regular business hours. However, many of the clinics are not certain of the courier pickup times, so staff place specimens in the box throughout the day. Physicians have noted a number of aberrant results, but consider those to be lab errors and whenever sufficient doubt warrants action, simply re-collect the specimen.

Explanation and Consequences

Exposure of specimens to heat and cold during storage and transit to the laboratory can affect the quality of test results. Freezing of samples can lyse cells (hemolysis), increasing levels of intracellular metabolites, such as potassium and lactate dehydrogenase enzyme. Heating samples can enhance metabolism within blood cells and within the plasma, elevating a variety of enzyme activities and changing concentrations of analytes, such as glucose and pH, within the specimen. Overheating can also degrade certain enzymes and unstable analytes. Drop boxes for specimen pickup by laboratory couriers can introduce a significant source of error. If these boxes are not kept in controlled environmental conditions by placing them inside of a climate controlled building, then specimens can be overheated in the summertime, and cooled or frozen in the winter. Sunlight can leak into the boxes and degrade light-sensitive analytes such as bilirubin. Physician office staff, as well as specimen courier drivers, all need to be mindful of recommended transport conditions and ensure that specimens are stored and transported appropriately. If couriers cannot pick up specimens and ensure analysis within a reasonable time frame, then physician office staff may need to process the specimens by centrifugation, and separate and then remove cells from the plasma/serum portion of the blood sample to stabilize the metabolites prior to the next courier pickup.

Specimen Processing Errors

The technique and manner of specimen processing can impact the quality of laboratory analysis. Failure to separate cells from the serum/plasma portion of blood allows for continued cellular metabolism that leads to decreased glucose values. Exposure of specimens to air, or transport of specimens with bubbles through a pneumatic tube, can alter blood gas values. Vigorous mixing of blood prior to analysis can generate foaming, which can affect pipette volumes and also induce hemolysis. Laboratories need to consider the possibility of preanalytical errors and take steps to minimize these errors.

Case with Error

A large health system has several small laboratories under the management of the health system's laboratory administration. While visiting one of these laboratories, the medical director noted that the laboratory had just acquired new centrifuges. The laboratory manager is very pleased, as the laboratory can now utilize the same centrifuge to process specimens for chemistry and urinalysis as well as to prepare platelet poor plasma for coagulation testing. During the visit, several technologists have raised concern over the speed of the new centrifuge. While the centrifuge can process plasma faster, the spins generate more heat and seem to be warming the samples. One batch of samples was just completing centrifugation, and the director noted that the samples removed from the centrifuge felt very warm. They measured 45–50°C using an infrared thermometer after the 5-minute spin.

Explanation and Consequences

A preparation of platelet-poor plasma is defined at $<10 \times 10^9$ platelets/L. This sample can be prepared by centrifuging whole blood at $>1500 \times$ g for 15 minutes. Incorrect conversion of gravitational force from g-force to RPM can lead to the use of the incorrect speed. Centrifuging for too long also can lead to overheating of the specimens, induce hemolysis, and generate stress on the centrifuge rotor such that it presents a safety hazard to staff in the laboratory. All centrifuges have a maximum speed beyond which additional gravitational forces can generate frictional heat and stress on the rotor. Refrigerated centrifuges can help dissipate some of the heat generated by higher speeds, but cannot reduce stress on the rotor. The technologists in this laboratory incorrectly used the wrong rotor size to calculate the appropriate speed and time for centrifugation with their new centrifuge. The centrifuge was being run at nearly twice the maximum speed, which was the reason for the heat produced. After contacting the manufacturer, the laboratory decreased the centrifuge speeds, increasing the length of the centrifugation and succeeding in processing specimens without overheating.

STANDARDS OF CARE

■ The clinical need for a test cannot overlook the issue of correct specimen identity.
■ The integrity of the specimen from identification through collection, analysis, and reporting of results must be maintained.
■ If a sample with a labeling error is analyzed, the test results should be associated with a comment to warn those interpreting the results of the potential for a specimen mix-up.
■ Institutions must have a specimen labeling policy to determine how labeling errors will be managed.
■ When the identity of a test result comes into question after analysis, the laboratory should never move the test from one patient's medical record to another patient's medical record.
■ Specimens should be labeled in the presence of a patient immediately after collection to ensure that the specimen label matches the positive patient identification.
■ The laboratory should be directly involved in phlebotomy education to ensure that staff understand test requirements and preanalytical variation that can occur during specimen collection.

▩ A laboratory should provide recommendations for limiting the exposure of specimens to extreme environmental conditions and to delays during transportation prior to processing and analysis.

RECOMMENDED READING

▩ NCCLS. *H21-A4: collection, transport, and processing of blood specimens for testing plasma-based coagulation assays: approved guideline.* 4th ed. Wayne, PA: NCCLS; 2003:23.

2 Core Chemistry

OVERVIEW

The modern clinical chemistry laboratory is highly automated. Specimens are barcoded during collection, and usually arrive at the laboratory ready for analysis. In a high-volume laboratory, an integrated system of instrumentation and specimen tracks connect the analyzers, identify the tests required from the specimen barcode label, then centrifuge, aliquot, and perform the entire analysis without human intervention. This automation greatly reduces the possibility of previously common analytical errors such as mixing up aliquots, ordering incorrect tests within the laboratory, making dilution errors, and reporting results to the wrong patient. Even for low-volume laboratories, automation in the latest models of instrumentation detects interferences from hemolysis, bilirubin, and lipemia that can affect certain results on individual specimens. These analyzers flag results to be held by the instrument management system pending review by the technologist prior to release to the ordering physician. Automated control processes can detect other analytical issues (e.g., calibration errors, out-of-range controls, failed delta checks and critical value limits) and warn the technologist of potential errors.

Thus, automation on laboratory analyzers is an essential tool that enables the technologist to identify those specimens with unusual characteristics and specimens that need repeat testing or separate handling. This improves the overall quality of testing.

However, automated analyzers are not foolproof, and good-quality test results require quality specimens. Mislabeled and mishandled specimens, inappropriate collection and transport, and miscommunication and misunderstanding of protocols and procedures can generate erroneous results that are not detectable by automated chemistry instrumentation. Careful attention to specimen quality is required both within the laboratory as well as outside of the laboratory. Preanalytical errors in test ordering, specimen collection, transportation, and processing, as well as postanalytical errors in delivery and communication of test results, contribute to overall error rates that are related to laboratory testing. These errors remain a concern even for the most automated of laboratories.

PREANALYTICAL ERRORS

Specimen Collection Errors

The manner of specimen collection can impact the quality of test results. Collection of specimens through indwelling catheters presents a deviation from routine phlebotomy practice. Clinical staff are tempted to utilize intravenous lines, because lines provide direct access to the patient's circulation, minimize patient discomfort from additional needlesticks, and are easier for the staff since there is no need for additional equipment or localization of veins. However, collection of specimens through a line poses a risk of contaminating the specimen with whatever fluid and, possibly, drugs being administered through the line. In addition, use of indwelling catheters to collect specimens increases the risk of specimen hemolysis, the lysis of red blood cells within the sample, which can affect some test results.

Case with Error

The laboratory began to notice higher rates of hemolysis from samples collected in the emergency department (ED). Upon investigation, the rate of hemolysis from the ED was 5 times that of other inpatient units. The problem coincided with a change in the flexible catheter that was implemented in the ambulance and ED. This catheter is made from a plastic that is firm at room temperature allowing for easy line insertion, but becomes flexible at body temperature for increased patient comfort. The ED has a practice of collecting specimens through indwelling catheters whenever they are available to avoid additional patient needlesticks.

Explanation and Consequences

Clinical staff will take shortcuts, especially if intended to enhance patient care and comfort. Sometimes those shortcuts can create more problems than they intend to solve. In this instance, the flexible catheter is similar to a soft rubber hose. Flow is unobstructed in one direction (the direction into the patient), but when flow is reversed (out of the patient), the tube collapses and increased resistance in the lumen leads to sample hemolysis. The product package insert warns users against collection of specimens through the catheter, since the reversal of catheter flow will collapse the tubing and increase resistance. The ED had not followed the product recommendations in this case. Hemolysis rates decreased when staff stopped collecting blood samples through this product.

Red blood cells contain higher levels of potassium, lactate dehydrogenase, hemoglobin, and other compounds that can affect analysis of these analytes, necessitating specimen re-collection and ultimately delaying the turnaround time of test results to the ED. The intent to enhance patient satisfaction by collecting specimens through an indwelling catheter actually created more delays in this case and increased the number of specimens for repeat analysis.

> ▶ Blood banks sometimes offer free laboratory testing as an incentive to encourage blood donation. Prostate-specific antigen, thyroid testing, or even cholesterol and glucose levels

are commonly ordered in this setting, and specimens for these tests are collected at the time of donation. Tubes are filled after the initial venipuncture during the start of the blood donation, processed, and sent to the core chemistry laboratory for analysis.

Case with Error

A patient arrived to donate blood in anticipation of a future scheduled surgery. The patient's physician had ordered a basic metabolic panel and coagulation testing, along with thyroid function and other tests. As a courtesy, phlebotomists collect these specimens at the time of donation to prevent the patient from having multiple visits and needlesticks. However, on this occasion, the phlebotomist forgot to collect the tubes prior to start of donation and simply filled the specimen tubes from the blood bag after collection. Upon analysis, the laboratory results were found to be unusual with low calcium, prolonged coagulation times, and critically high glucose. Upon laboratory investigation, the specimen was suspected of being contaminated with the additive used to preserve units of blood for transfusion. Fresh specimens collected via standard phlebotomy technique gave clinically sensible results.

Explanation and Consequences

Blood donor collection kits are packaged from the manufacturer with the necessary preservative already added to the bag, and use of donated blood as a laboratory specimen risks contamination with that preservative. One component of the preservative is citrate, which chelates calcium ions, decreasing calcium levels and prolonging times measured for coagulation tests. Citrate counterions often contain sodium or potassium and can thereby affect electrolyte levels, while dextrose in the collection kit can affect measurement of glucose levels. While intended to facilitate patient care, shortcuts to routine phlebotomy can sometimes adversely impact the quality of test results. In this case, the patient only experienced a delay in receipt of results and the discomfort of an additional phlebotomy from specimen re-collection. However, such errors could lead to clinical errors in interpretation with changes in medical treatment if not immediately recognized by the laboratory or the physician who ordered the test.

Metabolites, proteins, drugs, and other molecules can be unstable in a patient sample. Glucose, for example, will continue to be metabolized by red blood cells and white blood cells in the sample during transport to the laboratory prior to analysis. This sample will have lower glucose results than the patient's actual levels at the time of collection. A specimen collected in the right collection tube with the right anticoagulant can stabilize the analyte for more accurate results. Fluoride and oxalate, for example, can inhibit glucose metabolizing enzymes and stabilize glucose in a specimen over longer periods of time compared to a specimen without the preservative. Different additives are identified by manufacturers with characteristic colors for stoppers on the specimen tubes. Red-topped tubes are plain tubes with no additive, while green-stoppered tubes indicate heparin, purple stoppers contain EDTA, and gray stoppers have the glycolytic inhibitors, fluoride and oxalate. Collection of multiple tubes during the same specimen collection can risk contamination of tubes with anticoagulant from previous tubes in the same collection.

Case with Error

An emergency medical technician (EMT) who recently started working for an ambulance company is transporting a trauma patient to the regional hospital ED. The patient is difficult to stabilize, and the EMT has to collect blood while monitoring the patient's vital signs and discussing the case with the ED physicians. The EMT has a challenge locating a vein in light of the patient's trauma, but eventually four tubes of blood are collected; a purple-stoppered EDTA tube for cell counts first, followed by a green-stoppered tube for a basic metabolic panel, and finally two plain red-stoppered tubes for additional chemistries if required. Upon arrival at the ED, the samples are delivered to the stat laboratory while the patient is moved into one of the trauma rooms. Within 5 minutes, the laboratory technologist calls the ED indicating that the potassium is elevated but the sample is not hemolyzed. Ionized calcium is decreased and coagulation tests are prolonged. The technologist suggests re-collecting the specimens.

Explanation and Consequences

The specimens appear to be contaminated with EDTA. Because specimen collection tubes contain different additives, there is a recommended order of draw during phlebotomy to minimize contamination of later tubes by preservatives from earlier tubes that can affect test results. EDTA chelates ions such as calcium, leading to falsely decreased values and prolonged coagulation times. EDTA is added to specimen collection tubes in the form of potassium EDTA that can lead to falsely increased levels of potassium in specimens. Specimens should be collected in the order of sterile tubes first, followed by blue-stoppered (citrate) tubes for coagulation testing, red-topped tubes with no additive, followed by green-stoppered (heparin), purple-stoppered (EDTA), and last gray-stoppered (fluoride/oxalate). In this case, mathematical correction to determine the true levels of these analytes is not possible. Therefore, all results are suspected to be inaccurate and will need to be re-collected. Staff interruptions can distract staff and are a primary source of errors. In this case, the EMT was new to the job and balancing multiple activities at the same time, including caring for the patient.

> Phlebotomy technique can affect the quality of the specimen and test results. Collection of a specimen at the wrong time or without required patient preparation can give misleading test results. Inappropriate phlebotomy technique can lead to hemolysis and the need to re-collect a specimen with a delay in results.

Case with Error

A laboratory director is experiencing a bout of food poisoning and goes to the ED for evaluation. In the ED, a nurse enters the exam room to draw blood. The nurse collects the patient's blood in a 50 mL syringe and then sequentially stabs the syringe needle into the rubber stoppers of 5 tubes under vacuum, pushing the syringe plunger to fill the tubes. Although ill, the patient cautioned the nurse against doing this because of risk of needlestick injury. The nurse snapped back with the statement, "Honey, I've been doing it this way for years! Don't tell me how to do my job!"

Explanation and Consequences

Phlebotomy practice as well as the general practice of medicine has evolved over the years. As new research reveals better and more efficient ways to operate, practice standards have changed to improve patient care and enhance both staff and patient safety. Risk of needlestick injuries has led to new infection precautions that include proper handling and disposal of sharps. Manufacturers of phlebotomy equipment have also developed self-retracting needles and tube holders to protect staff and facilitate specimen collection. Resistance to change is a key human resource challenge, and managers and directors should delineate current standards of practice and guidelines by which staff need to operate. In this instance, the patient discussed the issue with the ED physician and the nurse was counseled and removed from duty for retraining to current standards of practice before returning to the ED.

Specimen Labeling Errors

> ▶ In a highly automated laboratory, labeling and barcodes direct the processing, analysis, and reporting of results for each specimen. The specimen label is as important as the

quality of the specimen inside the tube. Errors in labeling can cause misdirection of the specimen within the laboratory, the wrong tests to be performed, inappropriate processing of the specimen, and reporting of results to the wrong patient. Incorrect labeling can also lead to loss or difficulty retrieving the specimen from storage for reanalysis or review at a future time.

Case with Error

A urine sample arrives in the laboratory by courier from an affiliate hospital with a stat request for osmolality, creatinine, and electrolytes. The specimen is labeled on the lid of the container, but the label on the side of the urine sample is blank. So, when the lid is removed, the container has no label.

Explanation and Consequences

A label placed on the lid rather than the container of a urine specimen provides little assurance that the specimen actually belongs to the patient, since lids and specimen containers can easily become separated and intermingled during collection and handling. A urine container should be properly labeled on the specimen container, before handing the container to the patient for collection, since an unlabeled urine specimen could sit in a common bathroom or on a cart next to other unlabeled specimens prior to labeling. This presents the opportunity for mislabeling with another patient's identification. Spending a few minutes upfront to properly label a specimen will prevent later delays or, worse, mistakes that report results for the wrong patient, for whom inappropriate medical action and harm may ensue.

▶ Systems that protect the integrity of a patient specimen throughout the entire testing process ensure that the label on the specimen matches the result reported to the medical record. When specimen labeling or patient identity is in question,

requesting re-collection of the specimen and not reporting a
result are better than reporting the result to the wrong patient.
Laboratory results become part of the permanent legal medical
record of the patient, so the ordering physician should be con-
sulted any time there is a question over the proper labeling or
identification of a specimen (or an aliquot of the original specimen) during the testing process.

Case with Error

A specimen arrives in the laboratory labeled with the patient's name and
birth date as Joe Smith, 1/5/1967. However, Joe Smith born 1/5/1967 is
not found in the laboratory information system, although there are patient
records with similar names and birthdates. One patient is Joseph Michael
Smith with birth date, 1/5/1967, and the other is a Joe William Smith
with birth date 11/5/1967. The technician entering the test requests into
the order entry system has two choices; create a new patient entry with
Joe Smith, birth date 1/5/1967 and no middle name, or choose one of the
existing records. A call is made to the ordering physician who becomes
very upset with the delay in the analysis. The technician explains that
the specimen was not labeled appropriately, as there is insufficient information to determine whether the patient is a new patient or an existing patient. The patient's formal name is Joseph Michael Smith, born
1/5/1967, but he goes by the name Joe Smith, which is why she labeled
the specimen as Joe Smith. Ultimately, in this case the specimen was
analyzed and results were reported to the correct Joe Smith's record.
However, along with the results, comments were added: "Interpret results
with caution. The integrity of the specimen labeling cannot be verified.
The specimen arrived with incomplete name and collection information,
and the specimen was analyzed at the request of the ordering physician."

Explanation and Consequences

Labeling mistakes can delay the analysis of a specimen, and can also
lead to errors in ordering, analysis, and reporting of results into patient's

records. The use of two unique identifiers is the minimal requirement for specimen labeling. Full name, birth date, medical record number, and Social Security number are examples of unique patient identifiers. Nicknames and common names, like Joe Smith, allow for mix-ups as there may be many patients with the same or similar name in the laboratory database. When there are questions about the integrity of specimen labeling, adding comments to the test result reflecting specimen management decisions alerts current and future caregivers to the problem. However, comments and disclaimers only provide a record of what occurred and do not ensure that medical action was not affected by an error.

ANALYTICAL ERRORS

Many types of mistakes can happen in the laboratory including errors in aliquoting, pipetting, dilution, calibration, and result entry, as well as those related to instrumentation. The analysis of liquid quality control samples is one means of detecting and preventing errors in the clinical laboratory. A control is a stabilized sample, analyzed like a patient sample, to determine if the test system is properly functioning. Results from control specimens that are within a target concentration range can verify the ability of the test system (reagent, analyzer, environment, and operator) to produce quality results with each batch of specimens. Clinical laboratory quality control principles were adopted from the manufacturing industry where products on a factory line are periodically tested to ensure that they meet specifications. As bottles of reagents sit on an analyzer, chemical activity in the reagents can drift and degrade over time. The analysis of controls verifies the stability of the test system and provides for reliability in the test results. However, when quality control specimens fail to achieve expected results, the laboratory must determine which component failed, correct the problem, and reanalyze the controls and patient specimens before releasing results. Patient results must only be released to clinicians when control results are acceptable.

Case with Error

Quality controls fail on an automated analyzer. Two levels of controls are analyzed daily, and the high control is outside of the target range by 3.5 standard deviations on the low side of the control mean, while the low control is also outside of the target range by 3 standard deviations low. Two standard deviations on either side of the mean is the acceptable limit for release of patient results. Staff repeat the control sample analysis, and again obtain unacceptably low results. Staff continue to repeat testing of the same sample with reagent, and on the fifth attempt find the high- and low-level control sample results just within 2 standard deviations on the low side of the control means. The technologist is satisfied that patient specimens can now be released and that additional analyses can continue.

Explanation and Consequences

Repeating the analysis of quality control samples until results pass acceptance criteria fails to acknowledge the purpose for analyzing controls. A control sample mimics a patient sample. If controls at two different concentrations both fail their target ranges and in the same direction of the mean, then the operator of that instrument needs to stop the analysis and troubleshoot the cause of the control failure. Control ranges are set with the expectation that only 1 in 20 analyses will randomly be outside of the target 95th percentile range; i.e., a 2 standard deviation limit. Control results outside of 3 standard deviations are less likely, representing a 1:100 chance of being random error, rather than a true deviation. The failure of two controls outside of 2 and 3 standard deviations, both on the same side of the control mean, should signal the operator that there is a system failure. With two more control samples also failing to achieve target ranges, there is even more of an indication that there is a problem with the test system. This operator continued to run the controls until they barely appeared in range, so that patient results could be released, according to policy. Low control value results could be due to either degradation of the contents of the sample, reagent degradation while stored on the analyzer, or some other analyzer problem that would generate poor result recovery, such as an incorrect pipetter calibration. Checking the expiration dates of the bottle of controls and reagents helps with troubleshooting. Since both controls demonstrated low recovery, the failure is more likely to be related to the reagents, calibration, or other instrument problem than the control samples themselves, unless both bottles were started on the same date/time and handled in the same manner. Operators need to take clues from the quality control samples and correct instrument problems rather than repeating testing in the hope the control specimen will at some point yield a desired result.

> Analytical methods are calibrated to be used for specific specimen types. Conversion from plasma and serum can alter the specimen matrix. Also, results may differ due to the preservatives that have been added when using plasma specimens. Laboratories verify method performance prior to offering a test in routine clinical practice by examining the assay precision, accuracy, linearity, and population reference ranges on a specific type of specimen. Laboratories must retain data from such studies. Whenever there is a question about assay performance, the original data can be used to document initial performance of the test system, assist in troubleshooting, and determine if there has been continued stability of instrument performance. Changing the specimen from serum to urine, or even to plasma to serum, requires a new evaluation of method performance since the test system may behave differently with different types of specimens.

Case with Error

A surgeon sends a sample from the operating room requesting bilirubin measurement on an abdominal drainage fluid from an abdominal catheter. The fluid is a black, tarry, viscous material, and the laboratory has never analyzed bilirubin on a body fluid, let alone drainage fluid from an abdominal catheter. The laboratory calls the physician who claims that the laboratory always does this analysis for him.

He asks if the technologist could just run the specimen and call him back with the result, saying that the result does not need to be in the patient's chart since he is only trying to determine whether the source of the fluid is bile or some other type of fluid.

Explanation and Consequences

If the laboratory analyzes the fluid specimen, they are required by the Clinical Laboratory Improvement Amendments of 1988 (CLIA) law to document the test result in the patient's medical record. Regulatory compliance practices dictate documentation of physician orders and results from completion of ordered tests in the medical record. The laboratory cannot just analyze the sample and call back the results without documenting them in the patient's chart. In this case, if the specimen is analyzed, the laboratory has no data to support the performance of the test system on that type of specimen, and results could be falsely elevated or falsely decreased. There would be no way to demonstrate that the test system response is linear with increasing amounts of analyte in this specimen matrix without conducting dilution studies. Another issue relates to the viscosity of the specimen so that the technologist would not know whether the specimen could be safely pipetted within the analyzer or if the specimen would contaminate the pipetting mechanism and affect other specimens. Cuvettes could also be contaminated, and there is no guarantee that the standard wash cycles on a chemistry analyzer would adequately clear the specimen to prevent it from affecting future specimens. Finally, if the specimen could be analyzed, how would results be interpreted? Since there is no reference range for abdominal fluid, a fluid that is not produced in normal patients, any result that is generated is uninterpretable. The physician would assume that a high bilirubin would indicate biliary source of the fluid rather than another organ, but if the test system demonstrated a high bias on this type of specimen, that conclusion would be false.

There are several reasons that laboratories should be careful about analyzing fluid specimens without prior validation of method performance. The latest College of American Pathologist Laboratory Accreditation Program checklists require inspectors to critically review body fluid validation data for laboratories that analyze fluids and other nonroutine specimen types. Laboratories should be careful about unusual test requests on specimen matrices that have not been validated, since reporting the result in a phone conversation and not in the medical record, or adding a disclaimer that the specimen type has not been validated, does not eliminate concerns regarding system performance, accuracy of results, and potential for clinical misinterpretation. Furthermore, clinicians may have insufficient understanding of the risks for misinterpretation of values that might be generated, focusing instead on a desired benefit from a test result.

POSTANALYTICAL ERRORS

> ▶ Critical or alert values are test results that represent a life-threatening situation, and require immediate and interruptive calls to a physician or clinical staff member that can take medical action. Unfortunately, for convenience, tests may be ordered by residents under an attending physician's name, and nurses may order tests for patients under a physician's name in a clinic setting. In these scenarios, the ordering physician of record may not have examined or even know the patient when he receives a call from the laboratory to accept and immediately act on a critical result.

Case with Error

A critical potassium value (2.4 mmol/L [reference range 3.5–5.1 mmol/L]) is called to an outpatient clinic after hours. The answering service responds, but cannot contact the physician of record and the physician on-call has no forwarding phone number. After several attempts to contact a physician who knows the patient, the patient's home is called. The patient has not been feeling well all day and was so weak he has not been able to get out of bed. The laboratory requests the patient to go to the ED and to let them know about the critical test result. The patient is seen in the ED and is discharged with a plan for follow-up with his family physician. However, repeated attempts to contact the original physician the next morning were also unsuccessful, and it is noted that the clinic is only open 2 days a week. The on-call service notes that the ordering doctor may be at an affiliate hospital that day. He is an eye surgeon who could be reached in an operating room. Once finally contacted, however, the physician refuses to accept the critical value. Despite ordering the test, he claims he was only ordering the electrolytes as part of a presurgical evaluation on behalf of another physician, and he disconnects the call after telling the laboratory to contact the other physician.

Explanation and Consequences

Laboratories commonly struggle with callback of critical or alert values to outpatient physicians. While hospitals are likely to have designated staff who can take clinical action at all times, outpatient clinics utilize call centers after hours, forget to activate call lines, and often fail with hand-off coverage to other clinicians who may or may not take responsibility in these situations. The laboratory is required by CLIA law to contact the ordering physician or clinical designee who can take clinical action. When the ordering physician refuses to accept a critical value, the laboratory has to contact other physicians who may know the patient and can take action (some health systems escalate critical calls to attendings, department chairs, and even the Chief Medical Officer of the institution), or call the patient to request that they come to the ED for evaluation. Some states, like Massachusetts, have adopted critical value policies where the medical board can take action against the licensure of physicians who fail to respond to critical value calls. However, most states do not, and laboratories need to actively educate health care providers who order tests and develop policies to remind them that they are responsible for tests that they order or are ordered under their name, and the need to follow up on the results of tests from patients associated with their name, even if it is an indirect connection.

STANDARDS OF CARE

▓ Phlebotomy through catheters should be reserved for those patients with truly poor vascular access, those at risk of bleeding complications from traditional phlebotomy, and other highly special clinical circumstance. If used, this technique must only be performed at the request of a physician, with full knowledge of the risks and benefits of catheter-collected specimens, and the person obtaining such a specimen must be fully trained in these special techniques and fully knowledgeable about the line. The specimen source must be indicated with the test result, and patterns associated with dilution or other problems must have comments associated with results so that clinicians can assess whether results match the findings expected clinically.

▓ At least 2 unique identifiers (full name, birth date, medical record number, or other identifier) must be used to confirm patient identification, and verify the information on the specimen label/barcode during specimen collection.

▓ Any failure involving control specimens must be fully evaluated to determine the cause, rather than assume that the failure was due to chance.

▓ Tests on body fluid specimens require specific method validation to verify adequacy of technical performance on that type of specimen. Test results on body fluids must not be reported verbally or disclaimed with comments, when a method used has not been verified or the system performance is unknown.

▓ Laboratories are required to immediately contact physicians with critical test results. Physicians must take responsibility for tests they order (or allow to be ordered under their name), and ensure follow-up on the results of all ordered tests.

RECOMMENDED READING

College of American Pathologists Laboratory Accreditation Program. *Chemistry and toxicology checklist*. Northfield, IL: CAP; 2012.

Department of Health and Human Services Health Care Financing Administration Public Health Service 42 CFR. Final rule: Medicare, Medicaid, and CLIA programs. Regulations implementing Clinical Laboratories Improvement Amendments of 1988 (CLIA). *Fed Regist*. 1992;57:7001–7288.

3 Therapeutic Drug Monitoring/ Toxicology

OVERVIEW

Drug analysis involves the testing of samples for medications, toxins, and poisons. The discipline of toxicology spans many medical applications of a drug test result. The test may be intended for forensic purposes where the result may be entered as legal testimony in a court of law. Such cases include criminal intoxication, driving while impaired, child custody, cause of death, workplace drug testing, and sports/athletic doping. Forensic testing requires samples to be collected under a chain of custody where the specimen handling from collection, transportation, analysis, and result reporting can be strictly documented. Chain of custody is a paper trail providing assurance of specimen identity and integrity in order to confirm that the specimen belongs to a specific individual, has not been tampered with, and that the associated test result can be legally defensible in a court of law. Toxicology testing can also be conducted for clinical purposes, such as in the acute care of an emergency department (ED) patient, prenatal care, rehabilitation, and pain management. Test results can be quantitative (numeric) or qualitative (positive/negative), and drug analysis can be conducted using a variety of specimen types including urine, blood, hair, nails, meconium, and gastric and other body fluids. Some toxicology tests are used to screen patients for broad classes of drugs, while confirmatory testing can accurately identify a specific drug or metabolite. Given the number of drug tests and medical uses for the results, ordering the right test for a given situation can be confusing. Part of the laboratory's role is to define testing options clearly, so that ordering clinicians can understand what test is appropriate in order to answer the specific medical question regarding their patients.

PREANALYTICAL ERRORS

Test Ordering Errors

Laboratories frequently offer panels of drug tests. This facilitates ordering of drug testing for the clinician, since staff can order 10 or more tests on a patient's sample with a single test selection. Manufacturers of drug tests also offer point-of-care drug tests in multiple test panel configurations for screening of patient samples without requiring complicated laboratory instrumentation. Such formats include urine collection cups with a panel of drug tests embedded in the cup. In this assay, the patient collects a specimen, and staff twists the lid of the container, inverts the sample, and reads the results several minutes later. While the concept of panel testing is convenient, the question arises whether the patient really needs all of the tests in the panel performed or whether panel testing simply increases the cost of care.

Case with Error

The laboratory of a small community hospital begins to offer drug testing at the request of the hospital's physicians. Drug tests are currently sent to a regional reference laboratory with a 2- to 7-day turnaround time, inconvenient for management of trauma, obstetric, and psychiatric patients. The laboratory implements a drug testing device that offers 9 tests in a convenient unit-use kit. The device tests for amphetamines, barbiturates, benzodiazepines, cannabinoids, cocaine metabolite, methadone, opiates, phencyclidine, and tricyclic antidepressants. The laboratory technologists simply pipette 3 drops of urine on a test cartridge, insert the cartridge into a reader, and results are produced 10 minutes later on the result printout. Results can then be manually entered to the laboratory information system and electronic medical record, with a call to the clinician as requested.

Shortly after implementing the test, staff noted a problem with the new test configuration. Orders for drug testing were accompanying the samples, but more testing was being provided by the new method than that for which the staff had written orders. Previously, orders for reference laboratory drug testing included a 7-test panel, but the new test kit contains 9 tests (adding methadone and tricyclic antidepressants). If the laboratory analyzes all 9 tests, methadone and tricyclic antidepressant results would not have a written order. If a patient is positive for methadone or tricyclics, the staff cannot legally report a result without a written order. If the technologist calls the physician with results, the physician will question why tests are being performed without orders. Test orders for single drugs present even more of a dilemma for the laboratory, as up to 8 additional tests in a 9-drug test panel are conducted that the physician did not request.

Explanation and Consequences

Federal Clinical Laboratory Improvement Amendments of 1988 (CLIA) regulations require a written clinician order for laboratory tests. Panels of drug tests create a dilemma unless the order exactly matches the analytical format. Positive drug test results in a patient's medical record can have ramifications for insurability, employment, and even child custody. In addition, to process claims, insurance companies require documentation of the patient's diagnosis and of medical necessity before reimbursement of laboratory tests. Orders for screening with a wide range of drug tests covering stimulants, antidepressants, sedatives, and other medications are not targeted to a specific symptom or diagnosis and often are not reimbursed in full by insurers. Selective orders targeted to the patient's condition and medical need are more efficient and less likely to generate false-positive results for unexpected or unwanted tests. Manufacturers of laboratory methods that offer panels of tests need to provide the option to select the tests individually. This allows only desired test results to be reported by an analyzer while unordered test results are suppressed even if they were performed. In this way, the technologist is not left with results that cannot be reported and the associated ethical issues.

> ▶ There is increasing demand for electronic medical records in efforts to improve the efficiency of health care and to reduce errors. The U.S. government has offered incentives to physician offices for adoption of electronic record systems. As clinics adopt electronic records, laboratory ordering and reporting systems for these clinics are also increasingly becoming paperless. Electronic interfaces can communicate test orders between the clinic and a laboratory, and these interfaces can allow test results to flow automatically into the patient's record as soon as they are available on the analyzers. Government incentives for adopting electronic records and increased demand have given rise to hundreds of different vendors offering information systems to physician offices. Interfacing between laboratories and these clinical information systems is complicated because there are so many different combinations of office system products for clinical information and laboratory information systems. In this environment, generic interfaces are often created for specific vendor combinations that can be modified for the individual clinic needs. Adoption of electronic interfaces between a clinical record and a clinical laboratory without implementing necessary customization (at additional cost) can lead to the availability of a wider test menu than was previously offered with paper requisitions in the physician office practice.

Case with Error

An electronic medical record system shared by several affiliated physician offices is being interfaced to the laboratory information system of a hospital core laboratory. The hospital adopts the standard off-the-shelf interface without specific customization to the physician office's test menu. During adoption, the programmers noted a number of tests that are not offered by the hospital laboratory, but are part of the standard interface. Since the hospital did not plan or budget for the expense of additional interface customization, these tests are simply added to the physician office test menu. The interface vendor has noted that building a wider group of tests at an early phase of development is simpler and less expensive than individually modifying the interface at a later time to add single tests as they are needed. So, an extensive menu of tests, some performed by the hospital and others that require send-out to a reference laboratory, becomes available to the physicians' offices when the interface is activated.

Shortly after adoption, the laboratory notes an increased frequency of orders for tests like Ecstasy and LSD (lysergic acid diethylamide) that have previously been rarely ordered by the hospital physicians. One case in particular was selected for consultation with the ordering physician by the laboratory resident on a 90-year-old grandmother being seen in the clinic for a neurological evaluation of potential Alzheimer's disease and dementia. Ecstasy and LSD were ordered as part of a 15-drug profile on this patient. When the physician was contacted, he claimed that there must have been some mistake and that he only requested the standard drug testing for this patient. Routine drug tests ordered at this facility for any neurologic patient include amphetamines, cannabinoids, cocaine, opiates, and phencyclidine. The physician claims that he did not order these tests for this 90-year-old patient. He just communicated the request to his nurse who had the office clerk key the orders into the new electronic ordering system. On further investigation, the office clerk heard the need to order drug testing, but did not know what drugs were needed. To be diligent, the clerk just chose to order all 15 of the available drugs that were displayed on the order screen.

Explanation and Consequences

Ordering systems and laboratory interfaces, whether paper or electronic, are intended to simplify the ordering process and help the clinician order the right tests for the patient and medical needs. Common tests and groups of tests that are frequently ordered are generally listed on the requisition or electronic menu screen, so the physician does not have to search an extensive database for individual tests by name. This menu is often customized by the physician based on disease prevalence and medical decisions that the physician typically sees in his or her practice. Ideally, tests should be selected based on pretest probability and how the result will be utilized for diagnosis/management/screening/confirmatory testing of the patient. Selection of tests at random or without deliberate choice based on relevant knowledge, skills, and abilities can lead to false positives or false negatives due to cross-reactivity, interferences, and other test limitations. These erroneous results can lead to more unnecessary testing and adverse events. Drug testing is no exception.

Ordering tests with low pretest probability of a condition is more likely to generate false-positive results that require follow-up or confirmation testing at additional expense. In this case, the patient is a 90-year-old grandmother with a possible diagnosis of Alzheimer's disease or dementia, and the probability that this geriatric patient is recreationally using LSD or Ecstasy is exceedingly unlikely without a supporting medical history. Thus, testing for such drugs in a low-risk patient represents an unnecessary expenditure of resources.

Effective communication is also required when translating verbal orders. Physicians may believe that communicating orders to an assistant saves them time, but confusion among support staff over specific tests occurs, especially when there is a large number of similar tests and test names from which to choose. When there is a limited available list on one side of a paper requisition, the chance of choosing the wrong test is much less than when selecting from a wide menu of tests in an electronic ordering system. This problem can be multiplied when rarely utilized tests display next to commonly ordered tests or are grouped, simply by the fact that they are all drug tests, for example. The physician should review the written order for correct translation prior to transmission, particularly when handing off the responsibility to another staff member. Ordering laboratory tests should not be viewed as a clerical function, as clinically sophisticated knowledge is often required for accuracy.

▶ Ordering the "right" test requires an understanding of the intended use for the result. For toxicology, results can be used for screening patients in the ED, managing prenatal care, or determining whether a patient is compliant with his or her pain management plan and rehabilitation program. In the ED, physicians are determining the cause of unconsciousness, anxiety, or altered mental status, while in the pain management or rehabilitation program, patients may actively be trying to deceive the physician in order to continue abusing drugs or obtain a refill for a narcotic prescription. Prenatal care plans to promote healthy fetal development pose possible legal consequences with risk of newborn withdrawal and possible child social services involvement with drug abuse. Thus, there are different requirements for testing, and drug tests are methodologically not all equivalent. Acute clinical management requires fast results when there may not be time for confirmatory testing, if it takes place hours to days later. On the other hand, clinical care with rehabilitation, pain management, or tests with potential legal consequences necessitate confirmation prior to reporting and medical action.

Case with Error

A methadone clinic begins to prescribe buprenorphine (Suboxone). Physicians want patients being prescribed buprenorphine to be randomly monitored for compliance as they are with methadone prescriptions. On the first negative urine test result, patients receive a warning and after the second negative urine specimen, physicians consider removing the patient from the program, as this may indicate that the patient could be selling the drug rather than taking the drug as prescribed. Some of the patients are under court-ordered rehabilitation, so that negative test results will be reported to their probation officer for possible legal action. Clinic physicians start ordering a buprenorphine urine test from their affiliated hospital. The samples arrive in the laboratory processing area, and client services staff treat the request as they would for any new laboratory test by searching the Internet to find a laboratory that can perform the test and sending the samples to that laboratory. Within the first week of ordering, the physicians start calling the hospital laboratory with complaints that all their patients are negative for buprenorphine. Repeated negative test results represent cause for removal from the program, so the clinicians want to make sure that there is not a problem with the testing.

Explanation and Consequences

Buprenorphine is an oral drug that is now routinely utilized for treatment of opiate withdrawal symptoms and rehabilitation. The oral formulation of the drug contains naloxone, which blocks the narcotic effects of buprenorphine if a pill is crushed and injected or inhaled. Buprenorphine is gaining popularity over methadone for managing opiate withdrawal because it has less risk of abuse. As buprenorphine arrived on the market, physicians started to request drug testing to ensure patient compliance with the prescribed regimen, and not diverting or selling the medication. Repeated negative test results represent cause for removal from the rehabilitation program, so the clinicians must be absolutely certain of the accuracy of test results. In researching the test, two problems were found. The reference laboratory cutoff for a positive test result for the assay was much higher than the cutoff for rehabilitation program patients. Second, the testing at the chosen reference laboratory was intended for identification of the parent drug in pills or powders rather than in a patient's urine. The client services staff had selected the wrong test for the clinical need of the physicians dealing with the patients receiving buprenorphine. Selection of the wrong test cutoff for a positive test, for a specific clinical situation, can generate false-negative results leading to removal of a patient from rehabilitation. Using the right test with the correct test cutoffs for the intended use of a drug test result is critical to correct test result interpretation and patient management decisions.

Specimen Collection Errors

Drug test results can have significant impact on patients' lives. Positive test results for opiates, cocaine, tetrahydrocannabinol (THC), amphetamines, and phencyclidine each could indicate that a patient is abusing street drugs. Patients with positive drug tests may be noncompliant with treatment program contracts and could have their opiate prescriptions stopped. Positive test results on patients returning from leave (for work or home visitation) from a supervised rehabilitation home could be evidence of continued drug use. Test results may lead to dismissal from a live-in treatment program and possible reversal of probation for patients under court-ordered rehabilitation. Positive results for employment testing or after on-the-job accidents could lead to refusal to hire, job suspension, firing, or liability lawsuits. In addition to all these potential consequences of a positive test, it must be understood that patients can adulterate or add substances to their urine sample after collection in an attempt to generate false-negative test results.

Case with Error

A urine specimen is being processed for analysis in a laboratory. The processor notes that the specimen has a green tinge and smells distinctly like lemon soap. The specimen container fills with bubbles when shaken that do not dissipate. The medical technologist questions whether the specimen is urine or whether something has been added to the urine such as dishwashing detergent or soap. The test is canceled due to possible specimen adulteration, and the physician is contacted to have the specimen re-collected.

Explanation and Consequences

Adulteration of specimens is an ever-present concern for drug testing laboratories. Drug test results can allow patients to legitimately obtain drugs through a doctor's prescription, stay in a required rehabilitation program, or meet the terms of employment. Patients with an addiction problem have motivation to continue drug abuse and will go to extreme measures in order to thwart a drug test. Patients may take diuretics or drink volumes of fluid just prior to a test in order to dilute drugs that may be present in the sample (dilutional interference) to below a limit of detection. A number of detoxification products are available for sale on the Internet that are intended to either diurese the patient (e.g., dilute out drugs and metabolites in the patient's urine), or provide substances to add to the sample after collection (an adulterant) and interfere with testing. Drug screening tests are often protein-based immunoassays and only positive screening tests continue on to confirmation testing by gas chromatography/mass spectometry (GC/MS). Strong acids, bases, or detergents, and many products under the kitchen or bathroom sink may be used. These adulterants are intended to denature the protein antibodies and prevent their binding in the test reaction or inhibit signal detection required for a positive test result. Adulterants can be carried into the bathroom in a purse, coat, or pants pocket and can be added to the specimen after collection. In this example, the adulterant was most likely some type of dishwashing detergent that had a green coloring and lemon scent.

No adulterant is, however, 100% effective for all tests, as testing methodologies differ. Some tests require an antibody to bind the drug in order to produce a signal; the greater the binding and signal, the higher the concentration of drug in the patient's sample. Denaturation or inhibition of the antibody/antigen binding in this test prevents an assay signal, which is interpreted as low drug concentration. If the signal is below the assay cutoff concentration for lower limit of detection, a negative result is reported. This would be a false-negative result because the sample could contain drug that cannot be detected due to the adulterant. However, there are other tests where the signal is generated by inhibition of antibody-antigen cross-links in the test reaction. Antibody in the reagent links drug-bound microparticles to form polymers that lead to sample turbidity. High sample turbidity is interpreted by the test as low drug concentration in the sample. Drug in the patient's specimen prevents antibody complexes from forming, decreasing sample turbidity, and this signals a greater drug concentration in the sample. Adulteration of samples associated with protein denauration with this method will lead to false-positive test results, since the adulterant acts in a similar manner to drug in the patient's sample, inhibiting antibody–antigen complex formation. Other tests, like point-of-care test cups and single-use kits, contain a separate internal antibody reaction that acts as a control. Disruption of this reaction invalidates the control, which is interpreted as an invalid result that must be repeated. Since the patient does not know which test method is utilized by any specific laboratory, a particular adulterant could generate a false-negative, a false-positive, or even an invalid result, depending on where the specimen is sent for analysis. Processing staff receiving samples in the laboratory must be observant for unusual sample characteristics such as smell, bubbling, and color that could indicate adulteration. Laboratories that conduct drug testing should at a minimum offer analysis for detection of sample dilution/adulteration by measuring urine creatinine concentration, osmolality, or pH. Specialized testing is also available by some laboratories that can detect common adulterants, such as nitrates or glutaraldehyde.

> Adulterants are not the only means that patients may use to thwart drug tests. Some patients may resort to substitution, the use of a synthetic urine or submission of another patient's urine as their own sample.

Case with Error

Several complaints were filed by teachers with the local police department about an unidentified man who was seen in the vicinity of an elementary school during recess over a period of several days. Police patrols of the area around the school were escalated, and the suspect was observed talking with students through a chain-link fence. When questioned, the suspect indicated that he was in a rehabilitation program that required regular drug testing. Since he was still abusing drugs, he was paying schoolchildren for their urine. The case was featured in the regional news media.

Explanation and Consequences

One cannot underestimate what motivated individuals may do in order to alter their drug test results. Patients can dilute a sample through use of diuretics, drinking volumes of fluids prior to the test, or even by adding water to a urine sample to generate false-negative test results. In the previous case, the patient added substances to the sample aimed at disrupting the mechanism of the test reaction to produce false-negative results. Substitution of someone else's urine is a third possible means of achieving false-negative drug test results. Internet suppliers offer both synthetic (dehydrated animal urine) as well as preanalyzed, certified negative human urine for sale. Physician offices and collection facilities should consider adopting collection policies that discourage or prevent the substitution of another person's urine as the patient's specimen. Patients should remove bulky clothing, coats, and jackets, and leave purses and other articles that may hide adulterants or urine specimens outside of the restroom. Bluing agents can be used in the toilet water reservoir in the event toilet water is used to solubilize a dried urine specimen. Collection facilities can further verify the integrity of a specimen by checking that the specimen temperature is within a range of physiologic body temperatures shortly after collection. Capping the hot water in the bathroom can discourage sample dilution or substitution of water for the patient's sample. Supervised collections where someone observes the patient providing the specimen can further discourage substitution, but observed collections also invade a patient's privacy and therefore are generally reserved for prisons or court-ordered drug testing. Supervised collections are not foolproof, as there are products available for sale that mimic genitalia, have a urine reservoir, and can even heat a fake urine specimen to body temperature. The use of specimens other than urine for drug testing, such as hair or oral fluid, can be considered, since these specimens are collected with less invasion of the patient's privacy. However, not all laboratories offer drug testing on oral fluid or hair, because the methodologies require validation and the specimen matrix presents test limitations not found in urine. Anytime there is the incentive for a patient to deceive a drug test, the laboratory personnel must take the necessary steps to support accurate results. A physician having a patient tested should select appropriate collection facilities, request testing for adulteration and dilution, and most importantly, assess the test result in conjunction with the patient's overall situation.

> ▶ Drug testing can be important in emergency management. Patients can present with altered mental status due to an organic disease process, such as low blood sugar or mental illness, from trauma, or, not uncommonly, a medication reaction. The physician must sort out what may be causing the symptoms and decide on a treatment plan. When drugs are involved, the laboratory must determine which drug among the thousands of possibilities the patient may have taken. Not only is the choice of specimen a consideration, notably urine versus blood, but also whether the analytical methods are sufficiently sensitive to detect the drug in question. Clues from the physical exam, past medical history, and the presence of pills or powders on the patient can narrow the list of potential medications and help determine the appropriate analyses required for identification of an unknown substance.

Case with Error

A patient is admitted through the ED of an acute care/trama center. His wife indicated that the patient has had a past history of drug and alcohol use, but has been abstinent for the past year or more. He was recently fired from his job, and was found by his wife running around their backyard shouting at trees. Upon physical examination, the patient had a large bag of dried mushrooms stuffed under his jacket. The bag was marked with a printed label, "*Amanita muscaria* from Washington State." The emergency medical technicians indicated that they found the drugs on the patient when taking vitals and starting the intravenous fluids, but placed them back on the patient upon arrival at the trauma center. The ED sent urine, blood, and the bag of mushrooms to the laboratory requesting specific analysis. This laboratory only performs tests for common drugs of abuse and serum alcohol, so the laboratory looked into sending the samples out to a reference laboratory for analysis. Pictures of the mushrooms were sent to the state Poison Control Center. The staff mycologist confirmed the identity of the mushrooms from the picture as *Amanita muscaria*. However, no specific tests are routinely available at clinical reference laboratories or even drug specialty laboratories for this specific type of mushroom ingestion. The patient had elevated creatine kinase (CK) and alanine aspartate transaminase (ALT), and the clinicians were concerned about possible delayed liver injury due to mushroom ingestion. He was admitted to the intensive care unit for monitoring with supportive care. The patient's symptoms resolved over the next several days. CK and ALT enzymes normalized, and the patient was transitioned to psychiatric counseling prior to discharge.

Explanation and Consequences

Sometimes, obvious clues are the best place to start when identifying the nature of an unknown ingested substance. In this case, the patient was in possession of dried mushrooms and was demonstrating unusual behavior. The ED needed to determine whether the altered mental status was due to the drugs or to another cause. The patient had a previous history of drug and alcohol use, which supported mushroom ingestion as an explanation of his symptoms. In addition, none of the common drugs of abuse including alcohol were detected in the patient's urine. The label on the bag of mushrooms indicated that the mushrooms were *Amanita muscaria*, and the state poison control center confirmed the identity of the mushrooms. Unfortunately, there are no specific tests for the many toxins found in *Amanita muscaria* mushrooms. Ibotenic acid and muscimol are the most biologically active compounds, and analysis for these compounds is not readily available from hospital or commercial clinical laboratories. Specific identification would require full-scan mass spectrometry or other specialized testing with the right chromatographic conditions for identification. Mass spectrometry is not available in many hospitals, and reference laboratory testing would require a conversation with the laboratory director to ensure that any specific testing would be able to identify the compounds in question. Such analysis would be delayed by specimen transport and analysis at a reference laboratory. Thus, acute management of ingestion must be handled symptomatically with supportive care until the drugs are cleared from the body, while monitoring for liver, kidney, and other organ complications.

This case exemplifies the complexity of trying to identify an unknown compound. A toxicology laboratory cannot test for every drug, and sometimes must rely on medical history, physical exam, and the physician's observations. With few specific antidotes available and limited ability to analyze for the range of available drugs, some drug ingestions and overdoses must be managed through supportive care without full identification of a specific unknown agent.

ANALYTICAL ERRORS

The number of significant figures in a test result can lead to errors of interpretation. Too much detail by reporting of results to the tenths or hundredths decimal place can give the clinician overconfidence in the precision of the method. Too little detail and rounding of results may give the impression that the laboratory's analytical performance is worse than comparative methods. The laboratory director must find a balance to represent the precision of the method and minimize the risk of physician misinterpretation of test results.

Case with Error

Immunosuppressant testing for tacrolimus/FK506 is conducted by immunoassay in a hospital laboratory. The therapeutic target for the assay (4.0–10.0 ng/mL) is close to the low end of the reportable range, 2.0 ng/mL. The method performance has an imprecision of 10% CV (coefficient of variation) in the low end of this range. This means that random variation of results for a sample with a concentration of 5.0 ng/mL is 4.0–6.0 ng/mL, and even greater at lower concentrations (e.g., a 1 standard deviation [SD] range at 10% CV for a level of 5.0 ng/mL is +/− 0.5 ng/mL, and a 2 SD range is +/− 1.0 ng/mL).

The manufacturer markets the test on an analyzer that can report to the tenth decimal place and it can also round the results to whole numbers. Based on the analytical performance, the laboratory decides to report results at the level of whole integer concentrations.

Clinicians utilize the results for several months without complaint. Then, a new physician joins the transplant team and complains about the laboratory's drug levels. He has transferred from a hospital where the tacrolimus/FK506 results were reported to the tenth decimal place, so he concludes something must be wrong with this laboratory that only reports whole numbers. He demands that the laboratory switch methods to a more precise analysis, like the method available at his former hospital, since he argues that he cannot adequately treat patients with a test result that does not report to the tenth decimal.

Explanation and Consequences

Both laboratories are utilizing the same methodology and since the analyzer and manufacturer are the same, they have identical technical performance. The only difference is that one laboratory is reporting whole numbers while the other is reporting results to the tenth decimal place for drug concentration. Random variation makes the tenth decimal place meaningless as the imprecision at the lower end of the reportable range spans several units. However, by reporting to the tenth decimal place, physicians had better confidence in the assay, assuming that this represented better precision. Laboratories need to understand assay performance characteristics in relation to biologic variation and assure physicians that reporting units are relevant to assay performance and adequate for decision making.

POSTANALYTICAL ERRORS

▶ Screening tests are utilized to rapidly identify potentially positive samples, amid a large number of negative specimens, for additional confirmation testing. Screening tests are generally automated assays that require little technologist involvement, compared to confirmation testing such as mass spectrometry, which is more labor intensive and costly. Screening tests gain efficiency for the laboratory by confirming only positive samples, rather than performing a confirmation level test on every specimen arriving with a request for drug testing. Screening tests have limitations and can demonstrate false-positive results from common over-the-counter and prescribed medications. Confirmation of screen-positive specimens is especially required whenever test results may lead to legal or medical action. Unfortunately, confirmation testing is not available in every hospital laboratory, so the turnaround time for a test result may be several days. For critical and emergent patient management, test results are needed much sooner. While physicians may request preliminary screening test results to allow for immediate clinical decisions, this can lead to incorrect interpretation of results and inappropriate patient management.

Case with Error

Some rehabilitation clinics have patients sign a treatment contract on admission acknowledging that a patient's continued abuse of drugs can lead to dismissal from the program. These clinics house patients overnight in supervised environments for managing withdrawal symptoms, to provide counseling, and to further limit access to street drugs during treatment. At advanced stages in such treatment, patients may leave the clinic for work and family visits. Random urine samples may be collected when high-risk patients return from visits in order to determine if the patients consumed any substances while away from the program. Delays in confirmation testing are inconvenient and create problems for counselors when patients are confronted with test results from several days prior. What the clinicians need are real-time turnaround of test results, preferably no more than a few hours after the patient returns to the clinic, so that appropriate counseling and action can be taken while the issue is still current. Out of necessity, the rehabilitation clinic wants drug screening results and cannot wait for confirmation test results to manage patient leaves and visits.

A clinic patient tests positive by immunoassay for amphetamine and phencyclidine. The patient had been compliant throughout treatment and was approaching the last 2 weeks at the inpatient facility with short visits away from the clinic as a transitional step back to unsupervised life at home. A urine specimen was collected when the patient returned from the last family visit, and screening results were available later that evening. The counselor visited with the patient and relayed the positive test results. The patient denied use of any street drugs. His medical history indicated a recent cold with cough and sinus congestion, and the clinic has been providing antihistimines, decongestants, and cough syrup for the patient's symptoms. Despite the patient denying use of drugs other than the cold medicines, the counselor, by contract, documents a first warning in the patient's chart. This warning limits the patient's future leave from the clinic and risks termination from the program for a second positive sample.

Explanation and Consequences

False-positive results are not uncommon with immunoassay drug screening tests. Cold medicines including ephedrine and pseudoephedrine can cross-react with antibodies in the amphetamine assay generating false-positive results, while cough syrup and dextromethorphan have been documented to cross-react with antibodies in the phencyclidine assay. Clinic counselors need to be familiar with common cross-reacting substances particularly when taking action based solely on screening results without waiting for confirmed test results. The clinic policies should address this possibility. The counselors could speak with the patient about the screening results, but hold action until confirmation results are available. Laboratories should meet frequently with clinics that are basing treatment solely on screening results to warn of test limitations and common cross-reacting substances.

Drug screen results are generally reported qualitatively and have defined cutoff concentrations that allow discrimination of positive samples with concentrations at or above the cutoff level from negative samples with concentrations below the cutoff. Samples that screen positive can then be analyzed by a more specific method, like mass spectrometry, that can confirm the presence of individual drugs or metabolites. The cutoff concentration in a confirmatory test must closely match the screening test cutoff concentration. Otherwise patients that are positive by screening may be negative by confirmation.

Case with Error

The physicians at a pain management clinic believe that the laboratory's screening method is missing the detection of opiates in some of the patients. The clinic is prescribing oxycodone, but some of the patients are turning up negative by the laboratory's screening test. The clinic has requested that the laboratory confirm all negative opiate screen samples.

Explanation and Consequences

This case presents two challenges. The first challenge is that antibodies in many opiate immunoassay tests do not detect oxycodone with the same affinity as morphine, codeine, or their glucuronide metabolites. Therefore, oxycodone may not be detected in the urine of patients taking prescribed oxycodone dosages. Alternative assays with better affinity for oxycodone are available, but do not necessarily detect the other opiates, including heroin, with the same sensitivity. The second challenge is that the sensitivity of the test and ability to detect a drug in a patient's urine sample depend on a number of factors: the patient's hydration status, ability to produce urine (problematic in renal failure), time since last dose, amount of last dose, chronic use versus single dose, and build-up of drug levels in the body. Thus, drug testing is not always reflective of drug intake, and at best, the use of drug testing serves as a deterrent against continuing abuse.

> ▶Critical values are life-threatening results that require immediate, interruptive contact of the ordering physician or their designee who can take clinical action. Laboratories are required by the CLIA to contact a live person and document that communication of the critical result took place with read-back (to ascertain the accurate comprehension of the verbal result). Critical value communication is generally documented with the test result in the laboratory information system (LIS) or electronic medical record (EMR). Contacting an appropriate person who is willing to accept a critical drug test result can be sometimes challenging.

Case with Error

A critically high trough value of 30 mg/L vancomycin (reference range 10–20 mg/L) was obtained on a sample at 10 PM on a Thursday evening. The specimen was collected in the afternoon, and the office of the ordering physician is closed with no answering service available. The laboratory tries several different phone numbers and ultimately passes the result to a pathology resident to contact the physician. The resident has similar problems and cannot reach the patient either. Since therapeutic drug levels are very dependent on timing of the specimen collection with respect to the time of drug administration, the resident decides to wait until morning when the physician's office is open.The resident presumes that the patient would not be getting additional doses of medication overnight. In the morning, the resident reaches the desk clerk at the physician's office who apologizes for forgetting to switch the telephone line to the answering service after hours. She transfers the resident to the ordering physician who refuses to accept the critical value. The physician admits that he did place the test order, but he only did this as a courtesy for the hospital who recently released the patient. The physician claims that he does not prescribe vancomycin and would not know how to treat a patient based on that result. This communication was documented with the test result in order to close the critical value call, but the connection did not resolve the clinical issue of the patient's elevated drug level.

Explanation and Consequences

Ordering physicians must take responsibility and follow up on tests that they order. The toxic effects of high levels of vancomycin are controversial, but toxicity from high drug levels has been linked to nephrotoxicity as well as ototoxicity in some studies. Thus, expected medical action would be to decrease the dose or re-collect the specimen in order to ensure the specimen was truly collected at the right time (sampled just prior to next dose) and confirm that the level was correctly identified as a critical value. Ordering on behalf of another physician does not relieve the responsibility associated with the ordering clinician. The laboratory often has problems reaching the right person when one physician orders on behalf of another, or when nurses and residents order using attending physicians' names. Fortunately for this patient, the resident contacted the hospital that recently discharged the patient to identify the treating department. An infectious disease physician had originally seen the patient and prescribed the drug, so that physician was contacted for follow-up and to make sure that the elevated level was not ignored.

> The controversy over whether vancomycin is linked to nephrotoxicity and ototoxicity alone, or in combination with other aminoglycoside antibiotics, has led to requests for stat testing from the laboratory. Clinicians often cannot obtain the vancomycin level results fast enough, and doses are being held for fear that the patient may be above the therapeutic range. Nurses are anxious to give the next dose, and want the drug level to confirm that the patient is not at an elevated level before giving the dose. However, in most cases, stat requests are unnecessary and the antibiotic doses do not need to be held.

Case with Error

A laboratory is receiving a number of complaints from the critical care units of the hospital. At least a dozen formal quality reports have been filed in the last month against the laboratory for delays in generating vancomycin results that are claimed to have impacted care of the patient. Nursing state that they cannot complete the physician's vancomycin orders until they know the drug level.

Explanation and Consequences

Requests for stat drug testing can be disruptive to laboratory workflow. Automated equipment processes specimens on a first-in, first-out basis in the order that specimens are queued. Stat ports are available on instrumentation, but use of a stat port moves those specimens before others, interrupting centrifuge runs and delaying the processing and analysis of other specimens. For some analyzers, use of the routine process for all specimens (stat and routine) is more efficient and provides sufficiently rapid turnaround times such that use of a stat port is unnecessary. Stat interruptions can actually degrade the laboratory's performance by affecting routine testing and creating delays for patients that may be equally critical (trauma, ED, operating room, etc.). Laboratories need to understand their automated processes, work to maximize efficiency, and minimize stat requests to those patients that truly urgently require the faster turnaround time.

There are really only a few instances where stat vancomycin levels are needed and a dose should be held pending the vancomycin result, for patients with impaired renal function and those that are at risk or clearly demonstrating symptoms of drug toxicity. Otherwise, the next dose can be given after collection of the trough drug sample, and future doses can be adjusted when the test results are available. Pharmacists can assist the laboratory in educating staff on the proper timing of specimen collection for therapeutic monitoring with respect to drug dosages, including when a dose needs to be held pending a laboratory result and when it does not.

STANDARDS OF CARE

▧ Physicians must be selective in ordering laboratory tests. Order what is medically necessary for a patient based on the symptoms and diagnosis. It is not appropriate to screen for an abnormality using large panels of tests. Manufacturers should provide the ability to select individual tests on their instrumentation instead of forcing panel configurations that encourage unnecessary tests.

▧ While grouping tests can facilitate physician ordering, panels of tests encourage overutilization of unnecessary testing.

▧ Laboratories must match test cutoffs for screening and confirmation tests for drug testing.

▧ Physicians and laboratories must consider the possibility of deception in drug testing. Patients can dilute, adulterate, or substitute their samples in order to generate false-negative drug test results.

▧ Laboratories must educate physicians on the limitations of drug screening tests and common sources of false-positive and false-negative test results.

▧ Results should only be reported to an appropriate number of significant figures. Assay performance should reflect technical and biologic variation and a laboratory must work with physicians to ensure that reporting format matches the true assay performance and medical needs.

▧ Critical values are life-threatening results that require immediate, interruptive contact of the ordering physician or a designee who can take clinical action. Ordering clinicians must be aware of this expectation and accept responsibility for patient management.

▧ Clinicians should rarely treat solely based on the screening test results for drugs of abuse. Drug screens can have false-positive cross-reactivities that require confirmatory testing by a more specific method to appropriately identify a specific drug and metabolite.

▧ Administration of the next dose of antibiotics, especially vancomycin, should rarely be held pending laboratory results, creating a false need for laboratory urgency when, for most patients, a dose does not need to be held. Pharmacists should assist the laboratory in educating clinical staff on the proper timing of specimen collection and dose administration for therapeutic monitoring.

▓ Laboratories must understand their automated processes, work to maximize efficiency, and limit stat requests to those patients that urgently require the faster turnaround time.

OVERVIEW

Point-of-care testing (POCT) refers to diagnostic laboratory testing conducted close to the site of patient care, outside of a central
or core laboratory setting. POCT is generally conducted by clinical
staff, such as physicians, nurses, emergency medical technicians,
and respiratory therapists, without formal laboratory experience
or background in laboratory testing. The advantage of POCT is
the speed at which test results can be produced, because a specimen does not need to be transported to a laboratory for analysis
and have results communicated from the laboratory back to the
clinician for medical action. POCT is conducted in a variety of
settings including operating rooms, intensive care units, physician offices, ambulances, and helicopters. POCT has even been
conducted on the space shuttle. An increasingly diverse menu
of rapid POCT is being marketed for testing, including blood
gases, electrolytes, glucose, numerous infectious diseases, drugs
of abuse, and hormones to assess fertility. These devices use
a variety of testing methodologies: biosensors, immunochro-
matography, and now even molecular diagnostics. POCT has his-
torically been perceived to be less reliable than core laboratory
testing because of extra challenges posed in ensuring operator
competence, quality control performance, appropriate analysis,
and test result documentation. POCT is often viewed by clinical staff as a distraction from patient care and a laboratory task
added onto an already overburdened nursing workload amid
managing patients and staffing shortages on the clinical unit. Yet,
POCT is not a threat to central laboratory analysis; it is an integral
part of patient care and an extension of the laboratory when a
centralized laboratory cannot deliver a fast enough turnaround
time for results. The laboratory should facilitate understanding of
medical need, how the test result will be utilized, and the various
options available for laboratory testing to meet clinical needs. The
laboratory is a resource for best practices and quality standards, and
can assist nursing and clinical staff in achieving reliable results, no
matter who performs the test and where the test is conducted. Optimal implementation, planning, procedures, and training strategies

that incorporate POCT into patient management pathways assist physicians in ordering the appropriate test for the patient while delivering reliable results that meet regulatory requirements.

IMPLEMENTATION MISTAKES

Failure to Recognize POCT Differences and Limitations

The inability to obtain a fast turnaround of test results from a central laboratory is often the motivation to implement POCT on the nursing unit. The laboratory is seen as the limiting step to discharging patients from an emergency department or moving patients through the hospital. However, all laboratory methodologies have limitations and unique interferences that can generate misleading test results when utilized on the wrong patient populations or on incorrect specimen types. These limitations need to be considered when choosing POCT over central laboratory methodologies.

Case with Error

An emergency department was experiencing complaints about patient backlogs and delays in triage. Glucose meters were implemented to determine patient glucose levels upon arrival and to facilitate triage by identification of hyperglycemia and hypoglycemia prior to patients being seen by the physician. Soon after implementation, some patients were noted to have significantly lower levels of glucose, 100–300 mg/dL, compared to follow-up testing by the core laboratory, which showed values of 500 to >1,800 mg/dL.

Explanation and Consequences

All glucose meters have limitations in the package insert, warning of the potential for low glucose levels in patients with hyperosmolar condition, with or without ketosis, and in patients with circulatory insufficiency due to shock, trauma, or blood loss. Universal screening of a patient with a glucose meter prior to history and physical assessment of the patient's symptoms fails to consider conditions that could lead to misleading glucose results. While universal screening of patients on arrival to the emergency department may be viewed as a strategy to facilitate triage, the use of glucose meters on inappropriate patient populations can lead to incorrect test results. In the situation of nonketotic, hyperosmolar diabetic conditions, glucose meters generate significantly lower glucose levels that do not match central laboratory methods until the patient is rehydrated and the electrolytes are normalized. Glucose meter results can be misleading for several hours to days after admission. Clinicians should be aware of these limitations when dosing insulin, fluid, and potassium replacement, not just in the emergency department but even after admission to critical care units. Clinicians should always question whether POCT results are reflective of the patient's symptoms and condition. If not, testing by a different methodology should be used.

Using POCT to Solve Overly Complex System Problems

▶ Why the test is needed and how the test result will be utilized in patient care decisions should be clearly defined before a faster result can be safely concluded to facilitate patient care. Measures of patient outcome should be benchmarked before and after implementation of POCT in order to determine if POCT improved patient outcome or simply complicated an already overly complex pathway of care. Sometimes streamlining the pathway of care is a better alternative than adding POCT with its associated burden of operator training and competency, maintenance, reagent storage, and documentation considerations to a clinical service that is already stressed.

Case with Error

A cardiovascular diagnostics unit requires assessment of patients' renal function and electrolytes prior to a procedure. Despite patients arriving 2 hours prior to the scheduled procedure, less than half of the laboratory results for creatinine and electrolytes are available from the central laboratory in time for the procedure to be performed as scheduled. This situation delays patient procedures and requires staff rearrangement of rooms and physician schedules. POCT is viewed as the solution to provide faster turnaround of results to facilitate patient assessment and ensure that patients meet scheduled procedure times. However, after implementation of POCT, fewer patients actually met scheduled procedure times than when the central laboratory was used for testing. The staff in the cardiovascular unit was forced to contend with maintenance, quality control, and other documentation of testing rather than attending to patients. POCT placed additional burdens on an already overworked staff.

Explanation and Consequences

Laboratory testing is frequently blamed for delays in patient care. However, sometimes the uncoordinated management of patients and ineffective communication on the nursing unit are the major contributor to delays. While implementation of POCT may seem to be an easy solution to obtaining faster test results, POCT does not solve communication problems or resolve management complexities. Reassessment of the patient care pathway on the cardiovascular unit noted several steps for improvement where movement of patients through the unit could be facilitated. Improving communication between the staff, managing open procedure rooms, the staff's use of walkie-talkies, and a "procedure board" (a map of scheduled procedures and rooms about to become open) in different procedure locations led to the greatest improvement in patients meeting scheduled procedure times. After streamlining the patient management strategies, the decision was made not to use POCT. Instead, specimens were collected soon after patient arrival, and turnaround time from the central laboratory was reduced through courier transport of specimens to a closer satellite laboratory facility in a neighboring unit instead of the central hospital laboratory. Thus, POCT alone does not improve patient outcome. The laboratory helped this medical unit better understand its coordination issues and work through different options on a trial basis.

Misunderstanding Regulatory Requirements

▶The United States Clinical Laboratory Improvement Amendments of 1988 (CLIA) law mandates licensure of laboratories testing human patient samples where the test results will be utilized to make clinical decisions. Even laboratories performing simple POCT such as pregnancy, urine dipstick, or glucose meter tests must apply for a CLIA certificate, pay a fee every 2 years, follow manufacturer's instructions, and agree to be inspected. More complex testing than POCT requires additional documentation of operator training and competency, quality control, maintenance, and written policies for patient preparation, sample collection, processing, analysis, and result reporting.

Case with Error

A resident working on the medical support team for a marathon race wants to utilize a hand-held blood gas and electrolyte device to test sodium levels of runners to assess hydration status. The resident borrows the device and cartridges for testing from the critical care unit of the hospital. A nurse on the medical team discovers the device and cartridges on a triage table and contacts the medical director of the race support team, questioning whether the test is authorized for use at the race.

Explanation and Consequences

A CLIA license covers laboratory testing based on the location of the service. One license can cover all testing in a hospital, because the hospital is typically considered to be located at a single address. However, testing performed at an affiliated clinic or separate location requires another CLIA license, since the clinic is at a different location and address. The resident performing electrolyte testing unknowingly created a "laboratory" at the marathon race by moving testing devices and reagents to that setting. Such testing requires a CLIA license, since an assessment of patients' hydration status will be made based on the test results, and patients may be administered fluid and electrolyte replacement. Thus, even though it is a 1-day event, this setting requires a CLIA license. Testing without a CLIA license carries the risk of severe legal penalties with the potential for suspension of the medical director's ability to bill Medicare for lab services for up to 2 years. The medical director of the support team for the race is responsible for supervising the activities of all staff at the marathon and for understanding federal requirements that govern laboratory testing.

CLIA regulations apply to clinical laboratory testing. CLIA applies to tests conducted within a formal laboratory or outside of a laboratory, in a satellite or point-of-care setting. CLIA also applies to clinical samples from U.S. citizens that are analyzed within or outside of the United States. The analysis of forensic specimens, nonhuman specimens, such as veterinary samples, and research testing are exempt from the CLIA law. However, tests that lead to a change in patient management or medical decision making are considered to be regulated under CLIA even if those tests are conducted as part of a research study.

Case with Error

The principal investigator of a research trial is submitting an application for review by the institutional review board (IRB). The study involves a trial of a new drug. Data from the trial will support market approval by the Food and Drug Administration (FDA). Most of the laboratory testing used to support patient management during the trial will be conducted at a CLIA-certified laboratory in the Midwest. Samples for molecular testing, however, will be conducted at the drug manufacturer's facility in Austria, a laboratory that is not CLIA certified. The molecular genotyping results will be used to create a database that will possibly guide the direction of future trials and drug dosing, but it will have no consequence in disposition of patients in this trial. Research nurses will be responsible for obtaining patient consent, performing history and physical assessments, screening the patients for pregnancy by using a kit provided by the manufacturer, and collecting, processing, and shipping all samples during the trial. In the research application, the principal investigator claims that the trial is exempt from CLIA regulations, because all testing is research and will be conducted as part of the trial. Thus, the principal investigator checks the box on the study application indicating that no support is required from laboratory personnel. The IRB approves the study with no review by the laboratory.

Explanation and Consequences

Research trials can be a confusing area for interpretation of CLIA regulations. When laboratory test results are utilized to make patient-management decisions, the facility must meet CLIA regulations regardless of whether the test results are part of a research trial or not. Screening tests such as pregnancy tests are often performed to determine if the patient can safely enroll in a trial, because drugs used in the trial may have teratogenic effects on a developing fetus. Conduct of the pregnancy test to the standards of good laboratory practice defined by the CLIA law is critical to the assessment of harm versus benefit for patients enrolled in the trial by the IRB. Even as part of a research trial, laboratory testing should be performed under a valid CLIA license in this case, since the clinician is making a clinical determination of whether or not to enroll a patient in the trial based on the result of the pregnancy test. The molecular genotyping test, however, will not be utilized by the clinical staff in this trial, and those results are intended for research in developing future trials and drug dosages. Thus, the foreign laboratory does not require a CLIA license in this situation, since that testing is for future purposes and will not impact the care of patients donating the samples. The application of the CLIA law to research trials requires a case-by-case review of how each of the tests will be explicitly utilized to manage patients during the trial. If test results will not be available to clinical staff or affect patient management during the trial, then the tests are research and are exempt from CLIA.

> ▶ Although method verification is only required for non-waived tests under the CLIA regulations, method verification is a good laboratory practice for all POCT regardless of the test complexity classification status. The site performing testing should know the method precision, bias, and reportable range of results, and verify the reference interval for normal results. Staff must be trained, competent, and capable of obtaining performance that meets expected manufacturer specifications as approved by the FDA.

Case with Error

A physician working out of a pain management practice wants faster drug test results. Currently patients present themselves for an appointment, and staff must wait until the next day to assess whether patients are compliant with their medication or potentially abusing illicit drugs. Offering on-site drug testing would facilitate patient counseling and assessment. Samples testing positive by the POCT method could then be sent out for confirmatory drug testing, and initial management could be based on the preliminary POCT results. The physician orders several boxes of drug tests to perform testing in the clinic, but the shipment will take a week or more to arrive. In the interim, a clinic nurse is sent to the local pharmacy to pick up kits that can be used to start testing patients while the office waits to receive its drug test kits.

Explanation and Consequences

This clinic intends to start laboratory testing on-site and will need to apply for a CLIA license before testing any patients. However, drug tests sold over the counter at pharmacies are simple, waived complexity tests, so method verification and other documentation of test performance are not required. Because management decisions will be made based on preliminary test results, the clinic should determine the correlation of results by its POCT compared to the laboratory that will be conducting the confirmatory testing to ensure appropriate test performance at the clinic. Simple drug tests utilize antibodies that can cross-react with a number of over-the-counter medications. So, positive POCT results may not be truly positive for a drug of abuse upon confirmation. On the other hand, such POCT tests could miss important classes of drugs due to lower sensitivity than the central laboratory method. A study to assess the correlation of clinic results with the confirmatory laboratory would reflect good laboratory practice in order to understand the performance of the test kits, despite their CLIA waived complexity status.

TEST ORDERING MISTAKES

Distinguishing POCT from Central Laboratory Tests

As a general rule, POCT uses different methodology than instrumentation found in the central laboratory. Some tests may generate comparable test results, but other tests may give quite different results. Clinicians ordering a test need to understand the differences between available test methods, and the test names need to be clear enough to ensure that the physician is ordering the right test for his or her patient. Simply naming the test "stat" or "POCT" does not ensure that the physician understands the appropriate specific test limitations or that the results will actually meet an intended medical use of the test. Laboratories need to work with their information technology and sales/marketing departments to review how tests are displayed on electronic and written requisitions, and to ensure that test-specific information is readily available to the ordering clinician, especially if multiple options exist.

Case with Error

A hospital recently implemented troponin testing by POCT to expedite patient management in the emergency department. Cutoffs for myocardial damage vary among different manufacturers, so the reference interval for interpretation of the POCT troponin is different (5-fold higher on average for the specific POCT test employed compared to the central laboratory troponin test). After implementation, the laboratory received multiple complaints from physicians who were confused as to why their patient troponin results were showing such great variability. For example, a patient would be 0.03 mcg/L by POCT (negative for the 0.05 mcg/L POCT cutoff for this test), but a follow-up test in the core laboratory on the patient/same sample would show 0.08 mcg/L results (positive for the 0.01 mcg/L cutoff for this test). One problem was in the ordering system. Troponin tests would show up on the same ordering screen with multiple options: "Troponin" = routine troponin performed in the central laboratory; "Troponin (Stat)" = troponin performed stat in the central laboratory; "Troponin (POCT)" = troponin performed in the emergency department. Sometimes physicians were ordering Stat troponin, thinking they were getting the POCT, and other times they were ordering the POCT troponin when they wanted the Stat test from the central laboratory. Physicians also were not clear on the differences in the cutoffs between the different tests. The confusion over interpretation of results from POCT and central laboratory tests posed a risk of discharging patients with myocardial damage.

Explanation and Consequences

The laboratory needs to review ordering systems whenever a new test is implemented. Four changes were put in place to resolve physician confusion over the new POCT troponin. First, the core laboratory troponin tests were renamed "Troponin – Lab (routine)" and "Troponin – Lab (Stat)" to separate lab tests from "Troponin (POCT)" in the ordering system. Second, a pop-up screen was set up for all POCT orders to remind physicians that the POCT may be less sensitive than central laboratory methods and to suggest that physicians consider confirmatory testing by the laboratory for patients with high clinical suspicion of acute coronary syndrome or myocardial infarction. Third, an interpretive comment was implemented for POCT results. Those POCT results below the 99th percentile of the reference interval ($\leq$0.02 mcg/L) are reported as "not detected." POCT results in the range between the 99th percentile of the reference interval (0.03 mcg/L) and the 10% coefficient of variation (CV) of the assay (0.05 mcg/L) are reported as "indeterminate." POCT results >0.05 mcg/L are reported as "consistent with myocardial damage." Implementing a gray zone or "indeterminate" range of results helps prevent patients who are close to a single assay cutoff from being positive by one test and negative by repeat. Similar comments and three interpretive ranges (not detected, indeterminate, or consistent with myocardial damage) were also implemented for the central laboratory troponin results. Finally, the laboratory partnered with the cardiologists and emergency department physicians to develop a patient management pathway of care. Patients presenting with chest pain would immediately receive an aspirin, have blood drawn for laboratory testing, and be set up for an electrocardiogram. Timing would also start for follow-up testing and further assessments based on preliminary results. If indicated, the initial blood tests would direct the physician to the fastest assessment test, a POCT troponin rather than the central laboratory test. If follow-up testing is required at 3–6 hours for initial POCT negative or indeterminate results, the physician is directed by the ordering pathway to the central laboratory test, which is the more sensitive test prior to an expected discharge (with patients discharged if both initial POCT and 3–6 hour central laboratory tests are negative). Once these changes were made, no further complaints occurred from the emergency department physicians. Integrating the specific tests into the pathways of care ensured appropriate ordering of the right test at the right time on patients presenting with chest pain.

Overutilization of POCT

POCT can facilitate patient outcomes, but only if staff are available to act on the test results. If the ordering physician is away from the unit, and the POCT results sit in a patient's chart waiting for review, the intended benefit of a faster result is lost. Overutilization of POCT is a risk, because POCT is convenient to use on the nursing unit. It is easier than printing specimen labels and sending samples off to a central laboratory. Overutilization of POCT can be costly to hospitals because single-use tests are more expensive on a per-test basis than bulk reagents used in core laboratory testing. Without the benefits of improved patient outcome, performing POCT can waste both financial and staff resources in time spent performing the test outside the laboratory and documenting regulatory compliance. The decision to perform a test at the point of care or to send a sample to a central laboratory should be based on how the test result will be utilized in the care of the patient. POCT has a place in emergent management decisions for rapidly changing conditions, but orders for future POCT where the result is not linked to immediate care decisions should be carefully reviewed.

Case with Error

A POCT manufacturer increased the cost of reagent cartridges for a hand-held blood gas and electrolyte analyzer. Faced with economic pressures to contain costs, the hospital reviewed its use of POCT. Comparison measures showed the hospital was one of the largest users of this analyzer in that section of the country, considering case mix and complexity of the health care system. Larger institutions with comparable patient acuity were utilizing significantly fewer analyzers and cartridges. The increased use of POCT was not demonstrating a comparable advantage in patient outcome.

Explanation and Consequences

Physician leadership discussed the statistics with staff and made changes to the electronic ordering system for POCT blood gas and electrolytes. First, a pop-up reminder was implemented in the ordering system. This pop-up window identified the hospital as a large consumer of POCT cartridges and provided staff with the relative cost of POCT compared to core laboratory analysis, encouraging staff to use the core laboratory except in critical cases. The pop-up window also educated users by providing recommendations for several situations where POCT was warranted: emergent care of critically ill patients where the physician is waiting for test results to take action, severely anemic patients with hemoglobin <8 g/dL, and patients with excessive blood draws (>10 tubes in past 24 hours) because POCT uses less blood than central laboratory analyzers. The second change to the electronic ordering system prevented orders in the future for POCT. Only one action was allowed for ordering POCT: Stat, collect sample now, and analyze specimen immediately. Future POCT orders, such as potassium 3 times per day for the next 3 days, were prevented in the ordering system. After these changes, POCT utilization decreased by 50%–60% without a noticeable shift in patient outcome. Despite cost increases from the manufacturer, the hospital was able to maintain the budget through ordering system changes that controlled test overutilization.

PREANALYTICAL ERRORS

Collecting Samples through Indwelling Catheters

▶ A majority of laboratory errors actually occur outside of the physical walls of the laboratory and involve preanalytical errors, such as errors in specimen collection, as well as postanalytical errors, such as delays in acting upon results and result misinterpretation. Quality test results require quality specimen collection. A POCT device cannot compensate for a poor-quality specimen. Indwelling catheters are a common source of specimen collection errors because they frequently involve fluid or drug contamination of the specimen.

Case with Error

A physician calls the laboratory to complain that the POCT analyzer is not generating correct results. His neonatal intensive care patient has a 205 mmol/L sodium level that is physiologically not possible for the patient's condition. This is the second specimen in 2 days that has generated these falsely high sodium results. The laboratory questions whether this specimen was collected through an intravenous (IV) line, and if the infant is requiring IV fluids. The physician is adamant that he saw the specimen being collected, and it was not drawn through a line. The laboratory suggests that the physician personally collect a new specimen from the other arm or limb (a heel-stick would be acceptable) away from the IV line. A drop of that sample would be tested on the POCT device with the remainder sent to the central laboratory for confirmation. No specimen was ever received in the central laboratory as follow-up to this complaint. A laboratory review of the patient's medical record showed the patient had a 139 mmol/L sodium result measured by the POCT analyzer on the fresh sample collected after the telephone call. The physician apparently did not send the remainder of the sample to the central laboratory for comparison.

Explanation and Consequences

Line contamination is always a risk when indwelling catheters are used to collect laboratory specimens. Physicians should question results that do not match clinical conditions. Since an IV line is infusing fluid into the patient, staff often considers this an easy port for collecting blood from the patient. Unfortunately, the fluid in the line going into the patient can dilute the specimen when blood is collected out of the line. This increases the risk for analytical interference (particularly for drug infusions), or can alter the level of an analyte particularly if that analyte is a component of the infused fluid (such as sodium measurement when sodium chloride is in the line). The practice of withdrawing a few milliliters of blood or 3–5 times the volume of the line before collecting the sample may not be a sufficient volume especially for larger molecules that may stick to the lines, like vancomycin and the lipids in intralipid infusions. Staff may also have difficulty judging the volume of the line, as catheters can vary in length and diameter. A good policy is to only collect laboratory samples from an indwelling catheter on the basis of a physician order (when the risk of collecting through the line outweighs the potential for harm to the patient from a standard venipuncture) and should be reserved for those patients with very poor venous access, limited circulation, and risk of bleeding. Such specimens should have a notation attached such as "collected through line" to facilitate troubleshooting if results are questionable. The laboratory should help troubleshoot questionable results and be a resource for prevention of phlebotomy and other preanalytical sources of error.

Use of POCT on Alternative Samples

▶ Off-label use of POCT can raise the CLIA complexity of a test to a high-complexity level. High-complexity tests involve those developed by the laboratory or tests where the manufacturer's instructions have been modified. High-complexity tests require additional method verification and performance documentation. Staff may not realize that changing the specimen type or the intended use of the test (e.g., from monitoring for a disease to screening for a diagnosis) can change the CLIA complexity of a test and the number of additional activities that must be performed and documented for regulatory compliance.

Case with Error

Staff in a hematology/oncology clinic would like to screen patients for occult blood in nipple discharge. As the clinic already has stool guaiac test cards, the physicians begin to use the cards for this purpose. The fluid is applied to the card, and developer solution from the stool testing kit is utilized to visualize the presence or absence of hemoglobin in the fluid sample.

Explanation and Consequences

The specific occult blood test utilized by this clinic is FDA approved only for use on stool samples. The developer reagent is also optimized for use on stool samples. Performance of the test on a different sample type such as a body fluid is unknown without conducting specific method validation studies. Matrices like gastric fluid may require a different test developer that includes a buffer to minimize pH interferences with the guaiac reaction. Effects from the sample matrix may influence flow of reagent within the sample, reaction with the guaiac chemical, and even color development. Because the clinic is using a different sample type than recommended in the package insert (an off-label use of the test), the test is now high complexity according to CLIA. Before testing patients, the clinic must validate test performance with the specific body fluid using the guaiac card, or alternatively choose a different methodology such as blood cell evaluation to detect blood in the sample. *Validation* is a process to establish the complete set of performance characteristics of the test, including clinical utility, as opposed to *verification*, which is a process to confirm that a laboratory can achieve comparable performance to manufacturer specifications. Validation requires more extensive examination of the test on a specific body fluid compared to verifying performance comparable to previously established performance specifications.

Quality Control Mistakes

Quality control is the analysis of a liquid-stabilized sample, in the same manner as a patient sample, to determine if the performance of the test system, reagents, operator, and device meet quality specifications. Quality control is analyzed periodically to ensure the reliability of patient test results. Newer POCT devices have computerized data management that facilitates the collection of operator identification, patient, and test information at the time of analysis, and links that information to the test result. Data management systems that can automate the documentation of test and quality control results greatly assist in compliance with laboratory quality regulations, as staff can forget to analyze quality control and continue to test patients.

Case with Error

Pregnancy and urine dipstick testing is performed in an outpatient clinic. This clinic has a historical problem with staff retention, and staff is constantly changing. As a result, the clinic management is in a perpetual state of retraining new staff and has issues with staff documentation of POCT quality control records. At least 2–3 times per month, one of the clinical staff forgets to analyze quality control samples or the quality control is analyzed but fails to test at the expected target ranges without staff troubleshooting the failure. Patient samples are nonetheless tested regardless of quality control performance.

Explanation and Consequences

Quality control is an essential part of good laboratory practice to document that the test system and operator are performing adequately. Incorrect results could be released without awareness that the results are inaccurate, unless routine quality control is performed. While the management at this clinic is trying to provide faster results for patient care, they are failing to consistently follow policy and document their actions and may be generating incorrect results. Manual POCT tests require much manual documentation. The process needs good organization and clear staff delineation of roles and tasks to maintain consistency of documentation. This clinic could benefit from implementation of POCT with computerized data management that automates some of the documentation tasks and helps staff with regulatory compliance. Some models of urine dipstick and pregnancy test readers remind staff to analyze quality control specimens and lock out testing if quality control has not been performed. These devices can also lock out testing if quality control is analyzed but fails to produce a result in the required range, prompting staff to perform troubleshooting. These features improve staff regulatory compliance regarding manual POCT by reminding them when quality control and other steps of a procedure are not completed. These features prevent patient testing until the necessary quality control procedure is completed and the results meet expected ranges. An automated reader can also be used to standardize the test timing and interpretation, reducing the possibility of inadvertent operator errors.

Sharing Operator Identification Numbers

▶POCT devices look simple, but there is no foolproof device. Like any laboratory test, errors can occur when devices are used incorrectly or testing is performed by untrained operators. Good laboratory practice requires the operator to read and follow the manufacturer's instructions. Inappropriate sample collection, poor timing, or result misinterpretation can lead to incorrect results. More complex devices requiring multiple steps for collection and analysis of specimens necessitate more detailed training and practice. CLIA regulations for professional use of a POCT device require documentation of initial operator training and, at minimum, annual checks of ongoing competency for CLIA moderate- and high-complexity tests. Keeping manual records for hundreds of operators can be time consuming and very challenging to maintain. Fortunately, newer POCT devices with computerized data management have the capability to lock out operators. This feature ensures that only trained and competent operators are providing testing. An operator must enter his or her own personal identification number before the device will unlock and allow patient testing.

Case with Error

A coagulation device with operator lock-out was implemented in a hospital to assist with documentation and compliance. Only trained operators can perform coagulation testing and each operator has to document annual competency to continue testing. The device data management program stores training/competency dates and warns operators 30 days prior to expiration to allow time for recertifying their competency. Operators that did not complete their annual competency were automatically locked out of testing by the data management system on their anniversary date.

One general medical unit had a particular problem with nurse competencies. The unit trainer recently moved to another nursing unit, and the nurse manager was too busy with annual budget preparation to follow up with staff competency records. Friday was the last day of the month and more than 60% of the nurses on this unit were locked-out of testing over the weekend. The following week, the laboratory POCT coordinator performed monthly rounds of each testing location and noted that the nurse operators were sharing identification numbers. Three of the coagulation devices had an operator's identification number taped to the front of the device with a note, "Use this number if you are locked out of testing." There were so may staff locked out of testing over that weekend that at times no one with current competency was available to perform testing, so staff started sharing identification numbers to access the device. The POCT coordinator met with the nurse manager and reported that, by regulation, the entire unit required retraining with a focus on security and consequences of sharing personal identification numbers.

Explanation and Consequences

Training and periodic checks on competency are an important part of ensuring appropriate test performance and quality results. Lock-out features provide checks that restrict testing only to staff with current training/competency. Overriding the lock-out feature allows anyone to operate the device. In addition, test results are linked to the operator identification number used during testing. If clinical/nursing staff analyze specimens under a single operator's identification, then all of the test results are tied to that operator along with any erroneous results and data flags/comments. For laboratory devices, sharing identification numbers not only allows unauthorized staff to operate the device, but also grants access to the patient identification and test results stored in the memory of that device. Sharing identification numbers for performing laboratory tests is comparable to sharing user names and passwords that allow staff access to other confidential information, such as medical records and patient history. POCT operators should be aware that sharing identification numbers for device access can breach patient confidentiality of results and such actions could subject them to the same disciplinary actions as would be used following inappropriate access of medical records.

ANALYTICAL ERRORS

Data Entry Errors with Patient Identification

> ▶ Data management provides a means of automating the data collection and documentation that ensure regulatory compliance. Each test result is linked to the date/time, serial number of the device, the operator, reagent lots, and quality control for the reagent and analyzer. With data management, there is a record of every test performed, successful or not, and error codes and action comments are captured when a test fails. Manual records inevitably miss the recording of some test results, and errors/repeated tests may not get documented. Despite its advantages, however, data management also creates the possibility for a new class of laboratory errors involving data entry mistakes.

Case with Error

Staff in a busy outpatient surgery center affiliated with a neighboring large health system conduct hundreds of tests at the bedside each day, including blood gases, electrolytes, glucose, and coagulation testing. These test results are all manually entered into the patient's record and, therefore, some of the results are never entered or are incorrectly transcribed into the patient's chart. The health system is moving toward adopting a total electronic medical record that will encompass inpatient and outpatient procedures, including the surgery center admissions. As part of the conversion to electronic medical records, a glucose meter with data management was implemented that could connect the surgery center POCT results to the patient's health system medical record through a data management system, and automate the currently manual transcription of POCT results. This was predicted to decrease the amount of labor spent on managing POCT data and improve the accuracy of data transcription. At the time of testing, staff enters their 3-digit operator identification number. The device unlocks to allow testing, and then staff can enter the patient identification number (7 digits), scan the reagent barcode, collect the sample, and perform the test. However, soon after adoption, several results each day were noted to be "stuck" in the data management system. Operators were repeatedly making data entry mistakes, and the POCT results often had an incorrect patient identifier attached to the test that prevented results from being linked to an active patient record.

A few weeks after adoption of the meter with the data management system, an incorrect glucose result of 290 mg/dL was posted to an adolescent's chart on the inpatient hospital unit. Insulin was administered by the covering nurse while the patient's nurse was out on lunch break. The patient became dizzy and collapsed, and the next fingerstick glucose read 32 mg/dL. The patient was administered orange juice and recovered without permanent injury. The patient was not diabetic, had never had a glucose concentration above 110 mg/dL in his record, and had no orders for glucose/insulin monitoring. The covering nurse had treated with insulin solely on the glucose level posted to the patient's chart, using the hospital's sliding insulin scale, without reading the patient's diagnosis and management instructions in the chart. Upon follow-up, the source of the glucose result was not from the adolescent but instead from a patient in the outpatient surgery center. This was determined from the device serial number and the operator identification linked to the test result. Staff had inadvertently entered an incorrect patient identification number that matched an active inpatient medical record, and the glucose result was electronically transferred to the wrong patient's records. The operators were counseled regarding the consequences of identification entry errors.

Explanation and Consequences

POCT results are sometimes handled differently by laboratory and hospital information systems if the test result is not directly from a physician order but is instead performed according to a broader protocol. In a protocol-driven situation, when a test is ordered and results are generated by the POCT data management system, the test is conducted and POCT results flow from the device to a data management system, onto a laboratory or hospital information system, and finally to the patient's electronic medical record. This is different from the usual process in which laboratory information systems hold pending physician orders until a sample is received and analyzed, and results are associated with that order.

A POCT data management system marries the test result from the device with a current patient identification number in the medical records system to create a POCT order, then reports and finalizes the result by placing it into the patient's electronic record. Incorrect entry of patient identification can cause POCT results to get stuck in the data management system, since in that case the test result is linked to a patient identification number that does not exist or is not currently active. Even worse, as in this case description, an incorrect patient identification entry could match a result to the medical record of another patient and report that result to the wrong patient's chart with the potential for inappropriate medical action and treatment. Manual data entry of multiple numbers poses the possibility of incorrect data entry, especially if the patient identifiers are more than a couple of numbers in length. A system that requires staff to manually enter several digits for each patient test is a setup for failure, due to the amount of testing and human data entry required. Automation can decrease the rates of data entry errors through the use of barcoding and the scanning of patient identification numbers from individual wrist bands.

Other Data Entry Errors

Data entry errors can occur with any step of the analytical process. Incorrect operator identification entry is detected by the device as an invalid or untrained operator attempting access and, if the feature is available, lock-out prevents patient testing. Patient identification errors, however, allow testing to occur, but the results become stuck in the POCT data management system. An invalid patient identifier tied to a test result that does not match an active patient medical record forces the data management system to search the admissions systems for that patient. If there is no match, the test result cannot be posted to the patient's record. Data entry errors can also occur in identification of control samples and reagent lots used for testing. These errors pose challenges to accurate compliance documentation.

Case with Error

Nursing staff in an intensive care unit were making an unusual number of patient identification errors. Manual entry was determined to be the cause, and barcoded wristbands were adopted to reduce the rate of data entry errors. While data entry mistakes did decrease, the errors were not eliminated by barcoding. Staff continued to make identification errors when:

- Patients were barcoded with another patient's identification
- Patients were barcoded with another hospital's identification number
- Wristbands were unreadable

In addition, the POCT coordinator noted a high frequency of the same patient identification number as a data entry error. Upon investigation, the number matched the lot number of the test strips in use for testing. Staff was scanning the reagent barcode when the analyzer was expecting a patient identification number. The staff also had a number of control sample mistakes. For example, the high-level control was analyzed when the device was requesting the low-level control to be analyzed.

Explanation and Consequences

POCT requires operator focus. A sequence of steps must occur in succession each time a test is conducted. Nursing staff, especially in an intensive care unit, are focused on patient care and can become easily distracted while performing testing. The proper sequence of data entry for POCT is (1) operator identification, (2) patient identification, and (3) strip/reagent lot number identification. Staff may mistakenly enter the strip lot for the patient identification, or analyze a low control solution when the device is waiting for a high control. Such results become evident in review of the data management system records when the high control is 50 mg/dL (low target) instead of 300 mg/dL (the high target). Data entry errors also occur when staff enter the correct data but in the wrong sequence. For the 3 data entries noted above, errors can also occur with failures to double-check patient identification against the information printed on the patient's wristband or by scanning old wristbands from previous admissions or admissions to other facilities (especially for the transferred patient) during testing. Operators must take a time-out from patient activities to ensure that the proper test, on the appropriate patient, is being performed in the correct manner, as recommended by The Joint Commission.

Blind Operators

Part of training is documenting that staff can perform the test and achieve a result that is within expected tolerance. However, training is more than simply orienting staff to the procedure. Staff must demonstrate that they can perform all ancillary tasks required to generate an accurate test result. Temperature monitoring, instrument maintenance, quality control testing, and result reporting/follow-up are all components of performing the test. Adequate performance of all steps of the testing process is necessary to demonstrate competency. This requires (1) direct observation of routine test performance; (2) monitoring the recording and reporting of results (including critical value communication); (3) review of intermediate test results and worksheets including quality control, proficiency testing, and maintenance records; (4) observation of instrument preventive maintenance and function checks; (5) assessment of test performance using previously tested specimens, internal correlation samples, and external proficiency testing samples; and (6) evaluation of trouble-shooting skills. All six of these criteria are now being reviewed by CLIA, The Joint Commission, and the College of American Pathologists (CAP) inspectors, as required elements of staff competency for CLIA nonwaived tests.

Case with Error

Review of identification errors on a nursing unit noted one operator that stood out from the other operators. This operator had 5 times the number of identification errors compared to fellow staff members. She had been retrained 3 times and continues to make identification errors. The POCT coordinator visited the unit to follow up with the supervisor, only to learn that the operator in question is legally blind. The supervisor sympathized that she needs to work, but has difficulty reading the numbers displayed on the device and keypad in order to enter and respond to the required steps for testing. The POCT coordinator asked if she should be performing the test. Because the operator had difficulty seeing the keypad and display, she could not report results and take required clinical action. The supervisor had not considered that aspect of this staff member's job functions and indicated that she would verify that the operator could perform the test appropriately. If not, she would send the paperwork to have her privileges suspended in the data management system. Two days later, the POCT coordinator received paperwork to suspend testing privileges for this employee.

Explanation and Consequences

Operating a POCT device is more than just applying a sample and pushing the keys. There are considerations for sample collection, application, maintenance, and reagent and control storage. Most importantly, staff must be able to achieve the correct result and be able to report that result for clinical action. POCT operators must be proficient in all of these steps to demonstrate competency. In this case, the operator could not adequately see the keys or device display, which limited her ability to adequately perform all of the required tasks for conducting the test. Other cases of limited abilities for staff to perform testing may include color blindness. The ability to discriminate subtle color change is required to visually interpret some tests like urine dipstick results. However, using an automated strip reader could allow staff with color blindness to continue to perform the test, as the visual interpretation of color changes is automated by the automated reader rather than visually interpreted. Competency is thus linked not just to a test, but to a specific device and the ability to operate that device properly.

Temperature Monitoring and Reagent Storage Errors

▶ Quality results require quality reagents. Test strips, kits, and control materials that are exposed to heat, cold, humidity, and other environmental extremes can degrade before being used in patient testing. Shipments of test kits can be exposed to heat during the summer and cold during the winter while sitting outdoors being loaded onto trucks and airlines for transit. Testing staff have no idea of the condition of the reagents upon receipt of a shipment. Thus, good laboratory practice dictates verifying the performance of kits within each shipment using previously analyzed specimens or specimens of known analyte concentration, such as control or proficiency testing samples. Once received, the responsibility for meeting manufacturer-recommended storage conditions falls upon the laboratory and staff within the hospital where the reagents will be stored. For POCT reagents, some storage will occur on the nursing unit. Refrigerated reagents and controls must be stored according to manufacturer specifications, and corrective action must be taken when kit storage does not meet those specifications.

Case with Error

The cardiovascular diagnostics area of one hospital is a shared space for multiple departments—cardiology, radiology, and endoscopy. Cartridges for coagulation testing are stored in a refrigerator and must be brought to room temperature for 30 minutes before use. The test cartridges are good until the manufacturer-stamped expiration date on the package if stored refrigerated (2–8°C), or for 4 weeks if stored at room temperature (15–30°C). Staff must monitor refrigerator and room temperatures on a log sheet, take action when the temperature is out of range by calling the laboratory POCT coordinator, and write a new expiration date on each cartridge when removed from the refrigerator. Compliance with these policies has been variable. Multiple days are missed during the month for temperature monitoring. Clinical staff fails to take action or call the laboratory when a refrigerator is out of range, and cartridges are stored at room temperature without updating the change in expiration dates.

Explanation and Consequences

The space and resources are shared by multiple departments, so that no single department feels ownership over the POCT process. To have reliable test results, however, all staff need to be accountable for the quality of processes. Temperature monitoring and dating of the cartridges seem to be the biggest hurdle. Manual temperature monitoring can be automated through continuous recording thermometers. Some are electronic and can be downloaded to computers in order to print temperature charts, while others record on paper and require a regular change of the paper charts. Either method requires a supervisor to review the charts and take corrective action for out-of-range temperatures, steps that may not always be done. If a large amount of reagents or a small amount of expensive reagents are being stored in a refrigerator, the site could further consider linking a continuous reading thermometer to an alarm system that requires someone to correct the problem before the alarm is silenced. Such alarm systems verify continuous temperature monitoring and better ensure follow-up for out-of-range results compared to manual logs and systems requiring staff to remember to take action.

The other problem, manual updating of cartridge expiration dates for cartridges stored at room temperature, could be facilitated by utilizing a date stamp (prevents hand writing each cartridge's date). Alternatively, the unit could decide to rotate stock every 3 to 4 weeks and just keep all of the cartridges at room temperature. By storing only 1 or 2 weeks' supply of cartridges on the unit at room temperature, the nursing unit would utilize their supply before they expire and remove the requirement for temperature monitoring of refrigerators. The room temperature storage conditions would still need to be monitored, but facilities and engineering sometimes keep records and monitor the hospital room environment. Those records may suffice for documenting the monitoring of room temperature and humidity, provided there is action when the temperatures are out of range, and someone has the means for contacting the lab when the environment goes out of range. The nursing unit will need a strong supervisor to manage the POCT process at this site, but by modifying operations from refrigerated to room temperature storage, the management process may be greatly simplified.

Failure to Follow Manufacturer's Directions

▶ POCT is challenged by the large number of staff involved in the process. In an average institution, there may be dozens of locations utilizing hundreds of devices with thousands of operators. The large volume of tests performed and the need to conduct the analysis the same way, from step A to step B to step C without variance, each time, poses a risk for error. With the pressures of clinical care and patient management, human nature will strive to gain efficiencies by using shortcuts to work around strict procedures and find ways to reduce the time staff spends on the test while maximizing time with the patient. No one intends for bad results to happen. Clinical staff simply do not understand the consequences of varying the procedures, or the effect that shortcuts may have on test results.

Case with Error

The POCT coordinator received a complaint from a nursing unit that the glucose meter was giving falsely low test results. The staff brought the meter to the laboratory where the meter was checked. Quality control was within acceptable range and review of the historical results in the meter showed no problems with quality control performance. The batteries were checked. The meter was clean and seemed to be in good working order. The POCT coordinator took the meter back to the unit and inspected the utility room where testing was being conducted. The room had a counter covered with absorbent pads to soak up spills. On the counter were open vials of test strips, and test strips were scattered across the absorbent pads. Some of the strips appeared to be new, while others were obviously already used. When questioned, clinical testing staff indicated that it was easier to dump the bottle of strips on the counter, because the opening on the test strip bottle was too narrow to allow gloved hands to remove an individual strip. When testing was completed, used strips would sometimes make it to the garbage but at other times, just landed back onto the counter. Testing staff were inadvertently reusing glucose test strips. Chemicals within the strip were consumed during the first test, and then after blood was reapplied to the same strip, the test gave lower than expected results.

Explanation and Consequences

Shortcuts can leave the results incorrect, as in this case. Procedures are written to be followed explicitly in order to prevent variation in practice and ensure quality results. This particular error was created when staff were trying to expedite the testing process. However, by exposing strips to air and reusing test strips, test results were compromised. After noting the potential for reused strips to generate a test result, the laboratory investigated devices from several manufacturers. Some meters issue an error message and prevent issuing a result from a reused test strip, while other meters give an incorrect result and provide no indication that the strip has been previously used. POCT programs need to emphasize the importance of following procedures and the consequences of taking shortcuts no matter how minor the change may seem, and users of POCT devices need to understand the basic principles of the testing process.

Taking Procedural Shortcuts

Procedural shortcuts can lead to errors. Shortcuts may occur within one test procedure, or they may occur across several tests; the latter type is more insidious to identify the cause and troubleshoot. Because POCT devices offer limited menus, several tests and devices are often employed at the same time on a nursing unit to meet medical needs. Having a single sample shared for performing multiple tests may create unpredictable types of errors.

Case with Error

The supervisor of a busy intensive care unit called the lab to complain that the unit's hemoglobin (Hgb) device was broken. The device was reading too high, above 20 g/dL on postsurgical patients with hemoglobins in the 6.5–8 g/dL range. The device and reagents were examined by the POCT coordinator, and the source of the problem was not detected. The complaint continued sporadically over the next several weeks, on different devices with different operators, until one day when the POCT coordinator was conducting the monthly unit inspections. The POCT coordinator noted an operator taking a shortcut for the hemoglobin procedure. Operators were trained to cut a piece of nonabsorbent cellophane or parafilm, and place a couple of drops of blood on the cellophane; this drop was then to be utilized to fill the hemoglobin test cartridge. Instead, the operator applied a drop of blood directly to a glucose (not hemoglobin) test strip and then filled the hemoglobin test cartridge from the blood remaining on the glucose strip. Glucose test strips function by absorbing the plasma, the liquid portion of blood, into the strip to mix with the chemicals and hold the cellular portion of the sample back. By sampling off the top of the glucose test strip, the cells in the drop of blood had been concentrated, which raised the hemoglobin results.

Explanation and Consequences

Staff should follow procedures, regardless of whether they need to perform multiple tests on different devices. Shortcuts can impact test results in unpredictable ways when procedures are not followed. Training must emphasize the need for strictly following the procedure and stress the exact collection, processing, and application of the sample to the device. Competency assessment should document staff's understanding and ability to perform the test as trained. Annual verification of competency is important in order to verify that each staff member is still performing the test as written in the procedure and that shortcuts have not crept into the process.

Sample Application Mistakes

Sample volume can affect a test result. Application of too much sample on a POCT pregnancy test strip, for instance, may flood the kit, dilute the antibody conjugate, and create problems with ability to detect and interpret the result. Too little sample may lead to failure of adequate specimen flow and not allow test and control reagents to react with their respective zones on the test. Staff may know and attempt to follow the proper procedure but take liberties with sample application, often because of a limited amount of sample or the medical urgency for the test.

Case with Error

Nursing staff in an emergency department are conducting urine dipstick testing using an automated reader. The correct procedure is to remove one dipstick from the storage vial, dip the test strip into the patient's urine, remove it, briefly blot the excess liquid by turning the strip on its side on absorbent paper or a napkin, insert the strip into the reader, and then press the start button. Results are printed out in 2 minutes after the reader scans all of the pads on the dipstick. Shortly after implementing this reader, the POCT staff started receiving complaints about the frequency of reader "errors." Operators were resorting to visual interpretation of the results because of the volume of reader errors. Upon investigation, the errors were associated with low-volume urine samples, <10 mL in a 100 mL specimen cup.

For these cases, operators were using disposable droppers to dispense the sample across the dipstick. Other operators were observed bending and rolling the dipsticks around the inside of the specimen cup in an attempt to wet the pads.

Explanation and Consequences

Changing the manner of sample application can affect test results. Urine dipsticks are intended to be dipped quickly into the sample. Dripping sample across the strip or bending the strip to apply the sample changes the manufacturer's intended mode of application, which can alter the way the sample interacts with the chemicals on the pads of the dipstick. When test strips are bent, the plastic backing gets a permanent curvature that causes the pads to misalign in the reader and generate an error. Glucose, pregnancy, rapid strep, and other POCT can all be affected by both the volume and method of sample application. Operators should be cognizant of the intended method of sample application and carefully follow manufacturer's instructions.

POSTANALYTICAL ERRORS

Infrequent Operators

Mistakes can occur with test interpretation, especially for manual, visually interpreted POCT. Staff should verify the method of interpretation and appropriate timing of test development. Lighting can affect color changes. Fluorescent, incandescent, and even natural sunlight can alter shades of color in the operator's visual interpretation of results. Storage of kits near a window can degrade colored conjugates within the kits, so tests should be protected from bright light by storing kits within the manufacturer's protective packaging until just before use. Over- and under-incubating of the sample can lead to false-positive and false-negative test interpretations.

Case with Error

A physician's office offers pregnancy testing on-site. The staff that routinely performs the test is on vacation, so the covering nurse is required to conduct the test. After applying the sample, the operator sets the timer and walks away. When the timer alarms, she attempts to read the result, but cannot remember if 1 line represents a positive or if 2 lines is a positive. She has only performed the test once in the past several months and cannot remember where the procedure manual is stored. The package insert is also not available, because operators discard the insert with the shipping materials upon opening new boxes of test kits due to the limited storage available in the office.

Explanation and Consequences

Operators that do not frequently routinely perform POCT can have difficulty maintaining competence. This is one reason for having written procedures that are readable and easy to follow. Staff who do not routinely perform a test should have their training periodically refreshed and competency verified before conducting patient testing. In this office, the nurse should have been checked for competency before covering for staff leaving for vacation. The procedure manual should be readily available, and covering staff should know where to find it. Package inserts should also be kept with the kits for any POCT. The package insert contained in each shipping carton should match the individual kits in that package. Manufacturers sometimes make important changes to the package insert that can affect the procedure, and this is done without notifying customers. The specific text and version dating of package inserts should always be compared against previous versions of the insert upon receipt of any new shipment of test kits. Changes should be managed prior to use of the test products, including updating written procedures and training.

Distinguishing POCT from Central Laboratory Results

▶ POCT is a different method from core laboratory testing, and the results will differ as well, even when the exact same sample is used for both tests. Each methodology has unique interferences and limitations. A POCT glucose result is therefore not the same as a result from another glucose method, and POCT sodium may not be the same result as that obtained by other sodium methods. Misinterpretation can occur if results from different methodologies are intermixed.

Case with Error

Patients in a hematology/oncology clinic require an estimate of renal function before receiving chemotherapy. Creatinine testing is performed on-site by POCT, but the POCT creatinine demonstrates a bias relative to central laboratory creatinine results. The bias leads to approximately 0.2–0.4 mg/dL positive bias in the clinically relevant range of 1.5–2.5 mg/dL. Pharmacists must change their clinical cutoffs compared to central laboratory testing in order to formulate the appropriate doses of chemotherapy. Otherwise, physicians would overcall the number and degree of patients with renal impairment if only the POCT result is used and not corrected for bias. A new electronic medical record is being installed in the hospital and affiliated clinics that would consolidate all laboratory test results to the same section of the medical record. The designers of the electronic record want to consolidate the same tests within the medical record, such that creatinine results from the central laboratory will be listed in the same row as POCT creatinine results under the single test name of "creatinine."

Explanation and Consequences

All test results are not freely interchangeable. In the creatinine example, POCT biases would lead to different chemotherapy dosages if interchanged with central laboratory creatinine results. Laboratory and hospital information systems need to distinguish among test methods and ensure that appropriate reference ranges consider method biases.

Reassessing Need for POCT

▶ The laboratory should regularly interact with the physicians utilizing POCT. As a rapid diagnostic test, POCT should be meeting an urgent medical need for results on the unit that cannot be met by central laboratory turnaround times. Even routine POCT should periodically be reassessed for need to ensure that the POCT test is truly required, particularly in light of ongoing improvements in central laboratory diagnostics.

Case with Error

Recent evidence-based guidelines for POCT were released that systematically reviewed the literature and made best-practice recommendations. Gastric occult blood testing was reviewed in these guidelines. No recommendation was made for or against the use of gastric occult blood testing with nasogastric tube placement or to guide antacid prophylaxis for intensive care patients because there was no evidence that the test improved patient outcomes. Based on these recommendations, the laboratory questioned the gastroenterology (GE) service of the hospital to determine the ongoing need for the test. Staff were using the test to guide nasogastric tube placement. However, the test card offers two tests, one for occult blood and the other for pH. The GE service indicated that the occult blood test was rarely useful, since the test is so sensitive that the trauma of tube insertion always leads to a positive occult blood test. However, the staff utilized the test card for gastric pH determinations. During nasogastric tube placement, a staff member tests fluid withdrawn through the tube to look for a shift toward acidic pH. This indicates that the tube has been placed in the stomach rather than the esophagus or into the duodenum. Use of pH testing reduces the number of x-rays required to confirm tube placement. Because pH paper is also available on the unit and less expensive than the combination occult blood/pH test, the laboratory suggests that the occult blood/pH test cards be removed from the units. Removal of the cards would reduce the labor involved in documentation, training, and competency for the staff, and would limit the chance of errors involving mix-ups between fecal occult blood developer and gastric occult blood developer solutions, similar looking reagents for two different tests. The test continued to be offered by the central laboratory for those rare occasions that someone needed a gastric occult blood test, such as during emergency department gastric lavage.

Explanation and Consequences

The need for POCT should be periodically reassessed. The laboratory is often placed in the position of supporting POCT without understanding how or why the test is being utilized in the care of patients. Tests like gastric and fecal occult blood testing have been used for years, and the new generation of clinicians has never questioned why, as the test was utilized in their training programs and their mentors have taught them something about the use of the test. Thus, the test becomes the standard of practice without any evidence to support improved patient outcome. With increased scrutiny of health care costs and labor shortages, the laboratory should facilitate reassessment of need and periodically question current practices, especially as more evidence is published.

STANDARDS OF CARE

▓ The laboratory must collaborate with medical staff to determine the need for POCT laboratory tests, turnaround times, and how the test result will drive further patient care decisions. The availability of pneumatic tubes for specimen transport, the proximity of the unit to the laboratory, and the specific instrumentation available in the laboratory all differ from one hospital to another. Whether to offer a test at the point of care is thus a unique decision for each facility, based on the overall needs and ability of the laboratory to meet those needs with traditional laboratory instrumentation.

▓ While the goal of POCT may be a common, shared reference range, differences between POCT and central laboratory results exist and must be considered when making medical decisions. Test orders and results for POCT and the central laboratory as well as other methods for the same test (e.g., blood gas analyzers) should be separate and distinguishable in the patient's medical record.

▓ Cost issues must not be the only consideration when POCT is requested. If a faster turnaround for POCT results leads to quicker discharge decisions, facilitates movement of patients through the health system, frees operating and procedure rooms, and opens beds for waiting patients, the additional cost of POCT may translate to better overall patient outcomes.

▓ The laboratory should be involved with POCT as a resource for promoting good laboratory practices, quality control, documentation, and regulatory compliance.

▓ Manual tests are more prone to errors. Data management should be utilized to improve regulatory compliance and to automate the documentation and transfer of POCT results to the patient's medical record.

▓ Written procedures, regular performance of quality control, and operator training/competency are all required components of good laboratory practice for POCT.

▓ Medical need should drive the implementation of POCT, and POCT should be included as a component of quality patient care where indicated.

RECOMMENDED READING

Clinical and Laboratory Standards Institute. *EP23-A: laboratory quality control based on risk management; approved guideline.* Wayne, PA: Clinical and Laboratory Standards Institute; 2011.

College of American Pathologists Laboratory Accreditation Program. *Point-of-care testing checklist*. Northfield, IL: College of American Pathologists; 2012.

Department of Health and Human Services Health Care Financing Administration Public Health Service 42 CFR. Final rule: Medicare, Medicaid, and CLIA programs. Regulations implementing Clinical Laboratories Improvement Amendments of 1988 (CLIA). *Fed Regist.* 1992;57:7001–7288.

Joint Commission. *2013 CAMLAB: Comprehensive Accreditation Manual Laboratory and Point-of-Care Testing*. Oakbrook, IL: The Joint Commission; 2013.

National Academy of Clinical Biochemistry. *Laboratory medicine practice guidelines; evidence-based practice for point-of-care testing*. Washington, DC: AACC Press; 2006.

5   Endocrine/Tumor Markers/ Special Chemistry

OVERVIEW

Endocrine testing concerns the analysis of hormones, peptides, and other compounds secreted by the glands of the body. Hormones can be proteins, like thyroid-stimulating hormone and parathyroid hormone, or smaller molecules like thyroxine or cortisol. Endocrine tests sometimes measure a hormone directly, but in other instances may analyze compounds affected by hormones. For example, in diabetes mellitus, primarily a disease of insulin deficiency or insufficient insulin action at tissue receptors, clinicians diagnose and manage the disorder through analysis of glucose levels rather than through direct measurement of circulating insulin levels. Endocrine tests are utilized to diagnose and manage disorders of the pituitary, thyroid, parathyroid, adrenal, ovary, testes, and other organs of the body. Due to the variety of different compounds related to endocrine function, testing for endocrine disorders involves a variety of methodologies. Competitive immunoassays that rely on the binding of hormones and metabolites to specific antibodies in the test reagent are often utilized. Glucose is measured by enzyme-specific reagents with colorimetric endpoints. Immunoassays and spectrophotometric assays can be automated on laboratory instrumentation, but more manual methods, such as radioimmunoassay and enzyme-linked immunosorbent assays, are also employed for analysis of hormones and compounds. Failure to follow basic laboratory practices with specimen labeling, collection, transportation, analysis, and result reporting can lead to test result errors. In addition, some hormones and compounds are unstable in patient samples, so appropriate specimen collection and handling are of particular concern to ensure accurate detection and quantitation of the amount of hormone in the patient's sample.

PREANALYTICAL ERRORS

▶Proper patient identification is paramount to good laboratory practice. The assurance of specimen-labeling integrity starts with the proper identification of the patient. Current standards of practice dictate the use of two unique identifiers as part of the patient identification process. These may include full name, birth date, medical record number, Social Security number, or other form of individual identification. As the first step in the testing process, the phlebotomist should check that the patient's name matches his or her identification, particularly when physician orders, test results, and insurance or other billing are tied to patient identification.

Case with Error

The laboratory completed the analysis of a patient's specimen from an outpatient clinic, and the laboratory information system flagged an unusual result for technologist review prior to finalizing the result for release to the patient's medical record. A positive pregnancy test was reported on a urine specimen from a male patient. Human chorionic gonadotropin (hCG) can be a sign of testicular cancer in men, as some cancers, such as seminomas, choriocarcinoma, and germ cell tumors, can secrete hCG. Upon calling the physician, it was discovered that the specimen was not collected from a man, but actually had come from a female patient. Further investigation revealed that the patient was unemployed, and her boyfriend had given the patient his insurance card so that she could have expenses for her doctor visit covered. Although ethnic and uncommon names can sometimes introduce confusion, as can sex reassignment surgeries, in this case, the doctor visit, test orders, specimen collection, and analysis were all conducted on the girlfriend. None of the office staff had noticed that the medical record and insurance information belonged to a patient of the opposite sex until the patient's test result was released.

Explanation and Consequences

Proper patient identification requires active verification of the patient's information. Simply asking if the patient is Bob Miller may get a positive nod from the patient's head, when in fact the patient doesn't speak English and may not in fact be Bob Miller. Active verification requires asking the patient "What is your name and birth date?" then verifying the response against the test requisition and specimen labeling information. Asking a patient to spell his or her last name and state date of birth can be another form of actively verifying information. However, just checking name and birth date on written documents is not sufficient, as other important information on the specimen label could be incorrect: date/time, medical record number, sex, or clinic/nursing unit. Any incorrect information can delay results, misdirect results to another patient's record, or have consequences with billing. Proper identification and verification of patient information is one of the first steps in the testing process and is a starting point for ensuring the quality of the specimen prior to receipt in the laboratory.

> ▶ The matrix of a specimen is affected by the type of anticoagulant used for specimen collection, and plasma is different from serum. Specimens can be collected in blue-stoppered

tubes (citrate for coagulation), purple-stoppered tubes (EDTA for cell counts), green-stoppered tubes (heparin for blood gases and chemistries), or gray-stoppered tubes (fluoride and oxalate for glucose analysis). All of these tubes will generate a plasma sample when centrifuged to separate the cells. However, not all of the anticoagulants are equivalent and will have variable effects on certain tests. Laboratories need to ensure that the specimen collection tube and specific anticoagulant have been validated for the particular test ordered.

Case with Error

A small community hospital has been hit by a nursing shortage. Existing staff have had to take on more tasks. In order to meet the clinical needs for morning and afternoon rounds, unit staff are now collecting blood samples. During the first day of taking on phlebotomy responsibility, a nurse is collecting specimens for routine chemistry and for thyroid testing. She has only ever collected blood gas samples in the past, so she intuitively selects two green-stoppered heparin tubes for the collection. While labeling the specimens, she notes that the thyroid tests require a red-topped tube. Having already collected the samples, she uncaps one of the green-top tubes and carefully pours blood from the green-stoppered tube into a red-stoppered tube, labels the sample, and sends it to the laboratory.

Explanation and Consequences

Collection of blood into green-stoppered tubes that contain heparin anticoagulant may not be acceptable for all tests. Coagulation tests, some albumin assays, and certain immunoassays can be affected by heparin. For this patient, the presence of heparin in the sample will affect the analysis of free T4 test, with interference caused by heparin physically binding to the thyroid hormone-binding globulin and displacing thyroxine from the protein. Thus, samples collected in heparin will have falsely elevated free T4 results compared to samples collected in red-stoppered tubes (no additive). Laboratories should be aware of test limitations and educate staff on differences among blood collection tubes and the potential for affecting test results.

> ▶ Diabetes mellitus is a disease of increasing concern in developed countries due to the prevalence of obesity and lack of exercise. Diabetes is a disorder of insulin deficiency or decreased insulin action at the tissues characterized by high blood glucose levels. Although diabetes is considered an endocrine disorder, diabetes is diagnosed and managed through the analysis of glucose levels rather than direct measurement of insulin concentration.

Case with Error

A clinical laboratory has noticed an increasing trend in the number of glucose critical values that need to be called to outpatient clinics after closing. Critical values are life-threatening levels that require immediate contact of the ordering physician or a clinical designee who can take medical action. The laboratory's critical values are low glucose test results below 40 mg/dL on specimens originating from the laboratory's affiliated outpatient clinics. Although the specimens are collected throughout the day, the critical values are being generated when the samples are tested during the evening and overnight shifts in the laboratory due to delays in transport of specimens to the laboratory. These delays are leading to physician complaints, because critical calls are interrupting physicians at night, despite the fact that the samples are collected in the clinic during the day. The physicians cannot understand why the glucose test results are not available in a reasonable turnaround time while the clinic is still open.

Explanation and Consequences

Glucose is unstable in a blood sample and will be metabolized until plasma/serum is separated from the cells in the sample. Delays in sample analysis can lower the levels of glucose through ongoing cellular metabolism, even after specimen collection. Glucose is estimated to decrease about 7.5% per hour in whole blood samples at room temperature. Metabolism of glucose in the sample is faster at higher temperatures, and in patients with leukemia due to increased white blood cell counts. In this case, the low glucose results are a consequence of delays in processing of the clinic specimens. Although clinic samples are collected from patients throughout the day, laboratory couriers only pick up specimens intermittently. The samples are then transported to the outreach processing center, prepared for testing, and shuttled to the laboratory for analysis. Delays between sample collection and analysis in the laboratory could be 6 or more hours, depending on the distance of the originating clinic. Glucose continues to be metabolized in the patient samples until the sample is processed to remove the cells that metabolize the glucose from the plasma/serum portion of the sample.

The laboratory has options for expediting the processing of clinic specimens. The laboratory could increase the frequency of courier specimen pickup trips. More frequent sample pickups could be implemented to ensure that specimens for glucose tests are processed within 2 hours to minimize glucose metabolism. However, delays may still occur despite more frequent courier visits because of traffic or weather conditions. Use of specimen collection tubes containing glycolysis inhibitors (e.g., a stoppered tube containing fluoride/oxalate) can stop or greatly minimize glucose metabolism in a specimen after collection. However, these inhibitors take some time to become fully effective, so metabolism may continue for an hour or more after collection, even with use of glycolytic inhibitors. An alternative and better option would provide the clinic with a centrifuge to allow initial processing of samples within the clinic. The clinic would collect samples in gel separator tubes and centrifuge the specimens on-site immediately after collection. Gel separator tubes facilitate processing because laboratory instrumentation can analyze directly from the original tube, eliminating the need to aliquot serum/plasma from cells during sample processing. The clinic would simply collect and label the sample, centrifuge it, and place the sample in the transport bags for courier pickup. The advantage of providing the clinic with a centrifuge is that samples could be promptly processed, minimizing delays that would decrease the glucose levels in the sample and compromise test results. In one way or another, laboratories must arrange for prompt processing and analysis of samples intended for glucose testing.

> The ordering of thyroid tests can be confusing. Laboratories can offer thyroid-stimulating hormone (TSH), thyroxine (T4), triiodothyronine (T3), free thyroxine (fT4), free triiodothyronine (fT3), T3 resin uptake (T3RU), free thyroxine index (FTI), thyroglobulin (Tg), thyroglobulin antibodies (TgAb), thyroxine-binding globulin (TBG), and thyroid peroxidase antibodies (TPOAb) in their thyroid function test menu. Clinicians must be familiar with each of these tests and their limitations to pick the right test to address their diagnostic questions. The desire to order more tests than needed is tempting, given the large number of available thyroid-related tests. Overutilization can lead to mistakes in result interpretation and can contribute to increased costs of health care.

Case with Error

A first-year resident is seeing a patient with symptoms of weight gain, dry skin, fatigue, and cold intolerance. Suspecting hypothyroidism, the resident orders laboratory testing. After signing onto the electronic ordering system and selecting thyroid tests, the resident is amazed to see the number of thyroid-related tests offered by the laboratory. He is unsure of which test to order, and does not want to interrupt the senior residents or his attending physicians, as this would reveal his lack of knowledge about thyroid testing. He chooses to order all of the available tests to ensure that the right test result is available for case rounds. The results come back with a slightly elevated TSH (4.5 mIU/L with an upper limit of normal range of 4.0 mIU/L) and normal fT4. All other thyroid tests were normal including TPOAb, except for a detectable amount of thyroid-binding inhibitory immunoglobulin.

Since thyroid-binding inhibitory immunoglobulin blocks TSH from binding to receptors, thyroid production is blocked, producing hypothyroidism. The resident diagnoses the patient with hypothyroidism and, due to the detectable inhibitory immunoglobulin, assumes that this must be the source of the patient's hypothyroidism. He suggests that the patient be worked up for autoimmune disease. Upon review of the case at rounds, the senior residents and attending correct the resident's assumption. The patient has mild hypothyroidism. The other tests provided incidental findings and were not needed, and the patient does not need further evaluation for autoimmune diseases. The patient should be seen in 6 weeks for another TSH test (and only that test initially) to confirm the elevated TSH result.

Explanation and Consequences

Laboratory overutilization is a concern because of the possibility of incidental results, and this often leads to additional testing to "chase" abnormal results, which increases the costs of health care. Consensus guidelines published from professional societies, such as the American Thyroid Association and the National Academy of Clinical Biochemistry (NACB), are available that provide specific best-practice recommendations for utilization of laboratory testing. The NACB has noted that euthyroid patients frequently have abnormal serum TSH and/or total and free thyroid hormone concentrations as a result of nonthyroidal illness or secondary to medications that might interfere with hormone secretion or synthesis. As clinicians can be confused by the variety of available thyroid-related tests, current recommendations are to use TSH alone as the first-line test for screening thyroid function. If the TSH is abnormal, then an fT4 result can usually confirm a diagnosis and point to other indicated tests. The many tests ordered in this case were unnecessary and misleading. In particular, the inhibitory immunoglobulin test is rarely ordered, and the detectable amount was apparently an incidental finding, since higher titers of antibody are required to be diagnostic of disease. Sequential testing is more cost-effective and provides better outcomes by minimizing the possibility of false-positive or incidental test results.

ANALYTICAL ERRORS

> ▶ Immunoassays incorporate specific antibodies to detect an analyte in a patient's specimen. However, there can be a number of interferences, including drugs and cross-reactive compounds that can affect test results. False-positive elevations in test results can occur from these interferences and cause incorrect test result interpretations and patient mismanagement.

Case with Error

The clinical laboratory receives a phone call from a physician questioning a patient's pregnancy test results. The patient is a 51-year-old menopausal female patient. She has had 3 serum pregnancy tests, each spaced a week apart over the past month. All of the hCG results are in the range of 40–50 mIU/mL (<5 mIU/mL is considered negative). The levels have not been rising as would occur in a normal pregnancy, and the patient had a negative urine hCG test result on her most recent visit. The physician is concerned the patient may have trophoblastic disease, such as a molar pregnancy or choriocarcinoma.

The laboratory retrieves the most recent specimen and reanalyzes the specimen undiluted and with a 1:2 and 1:4 dilution. The undiluted specimen generates a result of 46 mIU/mL, but both of the diluted specimens give hCG results below the assay limit of detection and are reported as negative. The laboratory next incubates an aliquot of the patient's specimen with heterophilic antibody blocking agent. The sample with the antibody blocking agent generates a negative test result. The laboratory suspects that the patient has a heterophilic antibody that is interfering with the hCG assay.

Explanation and Consequences

Heterophilic antibodies are human anti-animal antibodies arising against mouse, bovine, porcine, goat, and other animal immunoglobulins that interfere with laboratory immunoassays through the binding of antibodies in the assay reagent and give rise to false-positive test results. Heterophilic antibodies can arise from working with animals, eating meat, or even from environmental exposure to animal antigens. Injection of mouse monoclonal antibody therapy can also give rise to heterophilic antibodies. The presence of heterophilic antibodies is believed to be the source of many false-positive test results in 2-site immunoassays where the analyte cross-links 2 antibodies to generate a signal. The heterophilic antibody in the patient's sample acts to bind the 2 antibodies and generates a positive test result without the presence of analyte, which is the intended target of the assay. False-positive hCG results have led to clinical mismanagement, including surgery (hysterectomy), as well as radiation and chemotherapy treatment. Whenever the test results do not match the patient's condition, the laboratory and clinician should suspect the possibility of heterophilic antibodies. In these cases, the clinician can resort to urine testing because heterophilic antibodies will not be present in urine samples (unless the patient has renal nephropathy). For true results, dilutions of a serum sample should demonstrate "parallelism," where hCG in the sample is decreased linearly by the dilution factor and correction for the dilution should yield the undiluted test result. A lack of parallelism upon dilution is characteristic of an interfering substance, such as a possible heterophilic antibody in the specimen. Heterophilic blocking reagents are available that contain absorbing antibodies that block the action of anti-animal human immunoglobulins in the patient's serum. Incubation of a specimen with heterophilic blocking reagent, and subsequent centrifugation to remove problematic immunoglobulins prior to hCG analysis, can minimize false positives due to heterophilic antibodies. Another investigative option is to analyze the patient's specimen by a different methodology. Heterophilic antibodies tend to react differently in laboratory methods due to the variety of antibodies employed by manufacturers as components of their clinical assays. Therefore, laboratories should be aware of the possibility of false-positive test results due to heterophilic antibodies and recommend that physicians always interpret test results in conjunction with the patient's symptoms and clinical condition.

POSTANALYTICAL ERRORS

▶ The manner in which a test result is displayed can impact test interpretation. Clear display of test results is especially important when a series of specimens are collected at the same time or in close succession as part of a patient procedure.

Case with Error

A hospital clinical laboratory receives 36 samples collected from intraoperative adrenal vein sampling for aldosterone and cortisol analysis. The samples are labeled to identify the source of the specimens as right or left adrenal vein, as well as the number of centimeters within the venous catheter at which the sample was collected. All samples arrive together in a single transport bag, and are accessioned into the laboratory information system in preparation for analysis. Since the samples are not numbered with respect to order of collection, laboratory staff confirm the test orders and receive the specimens into the laboratory in the random order that they are removed from the transport bag. Since the samples were collected during the same procedure, all specimens have the same date/time of collection and are resulted after analysis to the patient's electronic medical record in the order they were received in the laboratory. The clinical laboratory receives a phone call from the ordering physician the next day, as she cannot understand the test results. The test results are displayed in the electronic medical record as a list of individual test results, each with an accompanying comment. Left and right adrenal vein samples are intermixed in the electronic record, and there is no sequence of display with respect to the distance within the catheter where the specimens were collected. The ordering physician is having difficulty reconstructing the sequence of samples collected during the procedure and their associated test results.

Explanation and Consequences

Aldosterone is an adrenal hormone that regulates salt balance and blood pressure. Overproduction of aldosterone is one of the main endocrine causes of hypertension. This overproduction can occur due to bilateral hyperplasia of the adrenal gland or due to a unilateral adenoma in a single adrenal. Sampling of blood from the adrenal veins can determine the bilateral or unilateral source of aldosterone production. Due to the complexity of the circulatory system around the kidneys, cortisol is also measured in the samples to confirm the collection of blood from the kidneys. The number of samples collected during the procedure can lead to clinical confusion when interpreting test results, because it is necessary to reconstruct the sequence with which samples were collected, with respect to the laterality and distance within the catheter inserted into the patient. In response to the challenges faced in interpreting test results in this case, the laboratory met with the physicians and developed a strategy to improve test result interpretation for future cases. The physicians developed a diagram of the circulatory system surrounding the kidneys. Samples will be numbered immediately upon collection, and the corresponding number entered on the diagram to show the distance and laterality of each specimen. This diagram will accompany the specimens in the transport bag sent to the laboratory, and the laboratory will accession each specimen in the order of their respective sequence. Test results will be entered on the diagram after analysis, and the diagram can be scanned into the patient's electronic medical record and faxed to the clinician. In addition, the test results will be displayed in the patient's medical record in the order that the specimens are numbered during the procedure. Use of a diagram and sequential specimen numbering greatly enhances the interpretation of test results with future procedures. Diagrams and visual tools assist the interpretation of test results, especially when multiple specimens are collected sequentially during a patient procedure.

STANDARDS OF CARE

▨ At least 2 unique identifiers must be used to confirm patient identification and verify the information on the specimen label/barcode during specimen collection.

■ Laboratories must arrange for appropriate specimen collection, prompt processing, and analysis of samples to ensure appropriate recovery of physiologic levels of unstable analytes in a patient's sample.

■ Overutilization of laboratory tests can lead to incidental abnormal results that can be misleading and lead to unnecessary follow-up with increased cost of health care.

■ Laboratories should be aware of the possibility of false-positive test results due to heterophilic antibodies and recommend that physicians always interpret test results in conjunction with the patient's symptoms and clinical condition.

■ Diagrams and visual tools assist the interpretation of test results especially when multiple specimens are collected sequentially during a patient procedure.

RECOMMENDED READING

National Academy of Clinical Biochemistry. *Laboratory medicine practice guidelines. Laboratory support for the diagnosis and monitoring of thyroid disease*. Washington, DC: AACC Press; 2002.

6 Laboratory Information Systems/Informatics

OVERVIEW

The laboratory information system (LIS) is more than a database that stores all of the test results generated by the laboratory. An LIS acts as an intermediary to the clinical information systems and electronic medical records (EMR) utilized by clinical staff to manage patient care. Most physicians do not have direct access to the LIS and never work within that system. In the clinical laboratory, results must be collected from the analyzing instruments by the LIS, managed, and transmitted for display to the physicians in the EMR. The interfaces between the laboratory analyzer and LIS to the final EMR can each be sources of error that laboratories need to consider. As data are electronically transmitted from the laboratory to the hospital and onward to other electronic databases and records in the physician's office, insurance companies, government agencies, and even personal health records, test names can be confused, decimal points moved, and comments misinterpreted. A new responsibility of the laboratory in the age of paperless records is verifying that the result is correctly displayed for the ordering physician and that it can be appropriately interpreted after it is transferred through the variety of electronic systems.

PREANALYTICAL ERRORS

Ordering Mistakes

▶ Test names typically convey both the purpose and utility of the laboratory analysis. Test names can also be confusing, especially when there are several closely related tests that differ in method limitations, sensitivity, or clinical application. The laboratory has a responsibility to clarify for both ordering physicians and information system programmers which test result is the correct one being reported. Misleading test names can cause the wrong test to be ordered and lead to specimen re-collection, repeat testing, result corrections, and duplicate ordering on an individual or, worse, systematically throughout a health care system.

Case with Error

A laboratory is starting to offer high-sensitivity C-reactive protein (CRP) for cardiac risk assessment. This test has been approved by the United States Food and Drug Administration (FDA) for the specific indication of cardiac risk by selective manufacturers. There are other CRP assays on the market, but they do not carry this indication. The laboratory currently offers CRP as an inflammatory marker of sepsis in children, but the range of this test is much higher than the new, high-sensitivity CRP test, which provides values at a much lower range. The laboratory manager is submitting a form to add the new test to the LIS system, but clinicians will need to distinguish between the two different CRP tests, both when ordering the test and when reviewing and interpreting results. What is an appropriate name that would distinguish the different indications for these two tests—CRP versus high-sensitivity CRP? Would physicians know the difference from the name? Will the pediatricians start ordering high-sensitivity CRP thinking that they could possibly detect infections at an earlier stage using the high-sensitivity CRP test? The laboratory could call the test cardiac CRP, to discriminate the cardiac application of the test from the standard CRP, but should the current CRP name also be changed, possibly to pediatric CRP, sepsis CRP, or some other name? A decision was made to name it the high-sensitivity CRP test.

Explanation and Consequences

Laboratory test naming conventions can be challenging. In this case, the laboratory is faced with creating a new name for the high-sensitivity CRP test that will distinguish the different FDA-approved clinical indications of the test from the current CRP test. There is no right or wrong name, and the laboratory will need to work with the clinical staff to ensure that the name selected is optimal for the organization. Education of staff will be needed to announce the test implementation, define how the tests should be utilized, and how to order the different tests. One option is to create a new test for high-sensitivity CRP and keep the current test name, CRP, as physicians will still need to order the current test. But the two test results also need to be distinct and clear in the patient's record. Physicians must be able to understand the difference between high-sensitivity CRP and CRP based just on the name when reviewing patients' charts in the future. There are limitations with any choice of test names. If the laboratory also changes the current CRP name to pediatric or sepsis CRP, the laboratory risks confusing staff who require the current test. If a physician cannot easily find a test of interest in an electronic ordering system, staff will find the path of least resistance to order the test, which may be a paper requisition and handwritten test using any name or description they feel is appropriate. Thus, the optimal test name requires consideration of clinical operations and physician deliberation. Staff will require education during implementation. Furthermore, queries of the LIS to assess testing volume or for quality assurance studies may not capture data accurately.

Tests other than CRP present name challenges as well. Physicians have difficulty understanding which vitamin D test, 25-hydroxy vitamin D or 1,25-dihydroxy vitamin D, to order for monitoring their patients' vitamin D status and vitamin supplementation. This confusion often leads them to order both tests. Depending on the individual testing laboratory, physicians may get mass spectrometry results that separate four distinct vitamin D species: 25-hydroxy vitamin D2 and 25-hydroxy vitamin D3 from 1,25-dihydroxy vitamin D2 and 1,25-dihydroxy vitamin D3. Physicians may not know how to interpret these results. In this case, only the 25-hydroxy vitamin D test result is needed to routinely assess and manage a patient's vitamin D status, and the 1,25-dihydroxy vitamin D test should be reserved for patients with parathyroid disease, renal disease, or other endocrine bone disorders. Separation of vitamin D2 from vitamin D3 is not required and often confuses the result. Other names of tests often performed in the clinical chemistry laboratory that are confusing for ordering or interpreting include hepatitis antibody versus antigen, hemoglobin A1c for diagnosis versus management of patients with diabetes, and direct versus calculated LDL. Laboratories should consult with both physicians and LIS programmers to ensure that test names are displayed in the clearest manner in order to correctly identify tests in both the ordering and EMR systems.

> ▶ Test names can also be confusing in the order and result interfaces between electronic record systems. A physician may want a specific test and use one name on the requisition, but the reference laboratory performing the test may call the test by a different name or offer several tests with similar names. Mapping test requests in one system to specific tests on a menu in another system is part of the programmer's job when developing communication interfaces between different electronic systems. The processing staff in the specimen-receiving area of the laboratory must further determine the appropriate test to select when translating test requests and written requisitions as they arrive in the laboratory. Placing test requests over an LIS interface or selection of the wrong test because the correct name is not known to the ordering provider can be a source of error.

Case with Error

A physician at an obstetrics and gynecology clinic is screening a patient for alcoholism as part of the prenatal assessment. A urine ethanol is ordered along with drugs of abuse tests. Since the physician could only find a serum ethanol in the electronic ordering system, he uses a miscellaneous paper requisition and requests the urine ethanol test in writing. The processor receiving the sample sees two requisitions from this physician: one for routine drugs of abuse screening on an electronic order and the other for urine ethanol on a miscellaneous requisition. Since most miscellaneous requisitions are send-out tests to a reference laboratory, the processor aliquots the specimen. Upon searching the reference laboratory test menu for ethanol, the processor selects a gas chromatography volatile screen and sends the sample out. The physician's office calls the laboratory manager the next morning after receiving the drugs of abuse test results inquiring about the ethanol results. Unfortunately, the specimen was sent out for the wrong test from the reference laboratory; the gas chromatography volatile screen was ordered instead of the enzymatic alcohol available in-house. The ethanol result will be delayed, because the sample was sent to the reference laboratory. There is an aliquot in the laboratory from the drugs of abuse tests, but this cannot be reanalyzed for ethanol because it has been open to the air since the previous day. The cost of the test was higher from the reference laboratory, but the laboratory had to absorb the cost difference. The physician only needed a routine ethanol measurement in the urine sample and not the entire volatile panel, so the patient's insurance will not cover the difference.

Explanation and Consequences

Selecting the wrong test among a list of tests with similar names is a common error. Misunderstandings between an intended order and the actual order can occur in the processing area of the laboratory. In this case, the processor assumed the test was intended for send-out since the specimen was received with a written requisition. An LIS can help prevent ordering mistakes by providing pop-up reminders at the time of order, by incorporating order sets based on best practice, and by suggesting follow-up tests for abnormal results. However, an LIS can also create the opportunity for error by listing too many tests with similar names close together on the requisition/electronic order screen without providing enough information about clinical utility or methodology to distinguish between the tests. Thus, the error was more a system flaw than a mistake of the individuals involved. The selection options provided on the test ordering screen were inadequate to allow the physician to order the desired test on a urine specimen (rather than serum), and the system allowed the physician to bypass the electronic ordering system by using a manual requisition. Electronic ordering systems need to provide sufficient information to distinguish between available tests and facilitate ease of ordering.

> Electronic databases are created to facilitate both data entry and retrieval. An LIS can provide internal checks to warn of potential errors and caution the operator to verify the data before continuing. When the operator ignores a warning or the system allows the operator to bypass built-in safety checks, errors can occur.

Case with Error

The hospital laboratory receives a complaint from medical records. A parent received a bill for an office visit and recent laboratory testing on her child (Anna Natalie Smith, birth date 04/06/2008), but the child had not been seen by a physician in at least 1 month. However, a patient with the same first, middle initial, and last name but different middle name and birth date (Anna Nancy Smith, birth date 06/07/2008) had been seen. The Medical Records office sends the laboratory a written notice to correct the report.

Explanation and Consequences

Unfortunately, the laboratory cannot simply move results out of one patient's chart and into another patient's records. The specimen was labeled as Anna Natalie Smith and analyzed under that name. In this case, the original result was modified with a comment that the result belonged to another patient, and the patient's bill was credited. The result should not be removed from the patient's chart, since the result had already been reported and was available to clinicians prior to the billing inquiry. Additionally, the result should not be moved to the other patient's record, since there is now a question of mislabeling of the patient specimen at the time of collection. This error occurred because staff scheduling the patient selected the incorrect patient record at the time of scheduling. All procedures, the office examination, and laboratory testing associated with the visit were therefore reported to another patient's chart. This system's LIS offers an electronic warning during scheduling whenever there are multiple patients with similar names. The warning cautions the operator to double-check the patient's name and birth date, as a patient with a similar name exists in the system. However, the scheduler accepted the warning screen missing the birth date and middle name differences. Staffing was short that day, and the scheduler was busy entering information on this patient while two calls were waiting. The error was also not caught by the physician or the office staff during the patient's visit and specimen collection, since all of the paperwork had been generated by the office scheduling system and could have been caught by others. This case should caution staff to double-check at least two unique patient identifiers thoroughly with any patient interaction, particularly those with common or similar names, and to heed electronic system warnings that are intended to catch certain identification errors.

ANALYTICAL ERRORS

With electronic information systems, many tasks routinely conducted by technologists are now automated. Lipemia, icterus, and hemolysis, common interfering substances, are now detected by the instrument automatically. Specimen clots and bubbles can be discovered by pressure sensors in the instrument probes during analysis. Automated devices centrifuge, aliquot, and label aliquots based on the specimen barcode. In many ways, laboratory instrumentation has become so automated that technologists can sometimes forget what they need to do manually because the analyzer has been performing it automatically for a long time.

Case with Error

Samples with high levels of tumor marker CA-125, above the calibrated linear range, are automatically rerun at a dilution of 1:5. If a specimen has a value that is still above the linear range with auto-dilution, the technologist must manually dilute the specimen up to another 1:1000 dilution with normal saline. A physician called the laboratory after receiving unusual CA-125 results. Two patients over the past few weeks had lower than expected CA-125 results. Both patients were under treatment for ovarian cancer with a history of ongoing levels >100,000 U/mL, but the most recent results were in the 500–2000 U/mL range. Upon review of the original instrument printouts, two different technologists had reported the CA-125 results without correcting for the manual dilution.

Explanation and Consequences

Laboratory instrumentation has become sophisticated, and electronic data interfaces can transmit data directly from the analyzer to the LIS and the EMR automatically. Analyzers can even correct for test results elevated beyond the linear range of an assay using specimen repeat and auto-dilution. Specimens that are auto-diluted by the analyzer are automatically corrected for the dilution prior to release by the analyzer. However, when specimens are diluted manually by a technologist, the analyzer is reporting a result on a diluted sample. The analyzer does not know about the dilution that the technologist made manually, off the analyzer, so the technologist must correct for the dilution factor and manually enter the corrected result into the LIS prior to releasing the result.

This type of error has been termed "PICNIC," an acronym for "problem in chair not in computer," because the error was human and not a mistake in the computer, interface, or electronic communication. Since this error occurred with multiple technologists and had potential to recur in the future, even with operator retraining, the LIS reporting interface was modified to require the technologist to enter the dilution factor as well as the "uncorrected" instrument result. The LIS then calculates the final result and posts the result for the technologist's review prior to result validation and release. A delta check was also created to compare current results to previous test results, so that dilution errors, calculation correction mistakes, and data entry mistakes might be detected more often.

POSTANALYTICAL ERRORS

▶ Laboratorians and clinicians have different needs for data review within an electronic information system. Laboratory staff focus on individual test results and comments, while clinicians look for data trends in multiple analytes over time. Electronic information systems can display all test results chronologically, but data can also be displayed in a tabular form where test results for the same analyte are shown over time. Trends in results can more easily be followed in a tabular display across a row compared to scrolling through multiple pages of chronologically displayed full text results. However, there is no perfect means of displaying laboratory data. Viewing tables of numerical data poses a risk of loss of information. Clinicians want to review as much data on a single page or computer screen as possible, since this is more efficient than paging through multiple screens in the electronic record. Yet, cramming volumes of results in a table can risk loss of individual test comments and accompanying details with the potential for clinical misinterpretation if those comments contain significant information.

Case with Error

A first-year resident starting a critical care rotation is reviewing a patient's potassium results, and sees a value of 2.9 mmol/L in the EMR. The patient has had fluctuating electrolytes (potassium of 3.5–5.5 mmol/L) and some renal impairment (creatinine approximately 2.0 mg/dL) after hip replacement surgery 2 days prior, but none of the potassium values have been this low. The resident wonders if the patient needs potassium replacement. The result simply displays a red 2.9, indicating the value is outside the normal range, there is an asterisk, and "L" indicates that the result is low. Previous potassium values are displayed in the result table showing the fluctuating trend. No other comments are apparent on the table, just the numbers. The resident calls the laboratory before ordering a potassium bolus. The laboratory technologist indicates that there are result comments, "Note: Possible line contamination, interpret results with caution." Other analytes show abnormalities: sodium 125 mmol/L, chloride 95 mmol/L, glucose 489 mg/dL, hematocrit 22% (previous value 5 hours prior was 32%). The laboratory technologist describes how to retrieve comments from the electronic record. Users can move the screen pointer over the result, where a box will display with the result units and reference range. Right-clicking the mouse while hovering over the result will display a menu, and then the resident can select the "comments" option from the menu to display the comments. The presence of a comment or other important information is indicated on the result display with an asterisk next to the result. The resident noted that he thought the asterisk just indicated that the result was outside the reference range and thanked the technologist for the information on how to access important comments.

Explanation and Consequences

The display of results in an EMR can vary and displays sometimes can be customized at the level of individual provider. Clinicians need to understand how to interpret the results within the specific electronic record and display of their institution. The desire to display as much data at the same time provides for efficient data review but risks suppressing some of the information attached to the result. Important specimen details may be hidden leading to potential misinterpretation, unless the physician actively reviews test results for suppressed comments. These comments may need multiple additional keystrokes or actions to display. Requiring staff to actively seek out specimen comments, rather than passively displaying information with the result, poses a risk that staff miss those details. Better systems function by drawing staff attention to important details rather than making users work harder to find extra information. The more actions and time required by staff, the greater the risk of overlooking comments that are important in interpreting test results. Such comments may include "specimen hemolyzed" or "potential line contamination, interpret results with caution," and these may not be seen if additional steps are required to see them. The laboratory should ensure that clinical staff who view test results are adequately oriented to basic operations within the EMR so that comments critical to the appropriate clinical interpretation of the result are not missed.

> ▶ The display of test results for the ordering clinician is cru-
> cial to the clinical interpretation. The laboratory may think
> its role ends with the analysis and verification of a test result in
> the LIS, but physicians do not review test results in the LIS.
> Results must be transmitted to an EMR for the physician to
> see the result. Glitches can occur in the communication inter-
> face between the LIS and the EMR that can change the result,
> trim the comments, or otherwise alter the test result and lead
> to errors.

Case with Error

A physician office laboratory was recently connected to the affiliated hospital's LIS in order for test orders and results to electronically transfer between the facilities. The interface was validated by the
programmers at the time of installation to ensure that test results and
comments were transferring correctly. Several weeks later during a
visit to the physician office, the laboratory client service notes that the
potassium results are not displaying correctly. A decimal place error is
occurring such that a 4.0 mmol/L potassium result is being displayed
as 0.4 mmol/L. Staff indicates that the problem started a few weeks
prior. The result could not be right, so they just ignored the value or
corrected the decimal in their heads. No one called to complain, as
they assumed someone was already working on the problem as part
of the new interface.

Explanation and Consequences

Test result displays are not just an abstract quality concern, but regulated by law. The laboratory is responsible for ensuring that test results display accurately and with optimized visual formatting for the ordering clinician. A verified result from the analyzer has to successfully be communicated and translated across various interfaces through the LIS and onto possibly many subsequent links so that the physician can see the results. The laboratory must ensure that the result is displayed correctly for proper interpretation wherever viewed by the clinician caring for the patient. In this case, a decimal error led to the laboratory shutting off the interface until the programmers could troubleshoot and correct the problem. All previous results were reviewed and corrected. The source of the error occurred after an update to the laboratory's antivirus software. Sometimes any change to a clinical server, even as remote as software updates, can affect interfaces and data transfer at applications remote from the change. Office staff should not just simply ignore a blatantly incorrect display of results that are part of the patient's legal record. Staff must call for service to correct problems as they are identified.

> ▶ How a test result is displayed can impact test interpretation. The recent push for ultrasensitive or third-generation assays emphasizes the clinical desire for higher sensitivity for disease detection. While an analyzer may be capable of reporting to a hundredth decimal place, the question is whether the method performance can achieve precision at that level to make the hundredth decimal point number meaningful. Reporting a result to two significant figures can mislead a clinician to assume better performance than can be achieved by the test method.

Case with Error

A physician client of the laboratory calls to complain about the laboratory's test for prostate specific antigen (PSA). The physician's friend directs a laboratory, and the sales representative from that laboratory has just left information about a new, ultrasensitive PSA test that can report concentrations down to 0.01 ng/mL. Since this sensitivity would allow earlier detection of tumor recurrence after prostatectomy, the physician demands that all his PSA samples be sent to his friend's laboratory with the new ultrasensitive test.

Explanation and Consequences

The friend's laboratory was researched, and both laboratories are performing the same test. The current laboratory reports PSA to the tenth decimal place with a lower limit of the reportable range of 0.1 ng/mL, while the friend's laboratory where the physician wants the samples sent is reporting PSA to the hundredth decimal place with a lower limit of the reportable range of 0.01 ng/mL. While this appears to be a more sensitive method, and the laboratory has recently started promoting the assay as "ultrasensitive," the "ultrasensitive" test has an imprecision of 20% at a level of 0.10 ng/mL. A 2 standard deviation (SD) range would span 0.06–0.14 ng/mL. With such imprecision at the low end of the reportable range, a laboratory would have difficulty assessing levels <0.1 ng/mL (such as 0.01 ng/mL) with any degree of confidence. Thus, while an analyzer may be capable of reporting more significant figures in a result, in practice, an assay cannot reliably discriminate small differences in a test result when close to the lower limit of detection. Physicians can be misled by advertising without understanding the true performance of a method.

> Results can be changed during transmission over electronic interfaces. The integrity of data transmission needs to be verified on an ongoing basis to ensure correct appearance for the ordering physician. Errors can occur when data are changed, with an obvious potential for result misinterpretation.

Case with Error

The laboratory director receives a phone call from a gynecology office requesting results on 2 patients in their practice. Both patients are undergoing treatment for ovarian cancer and have high levels of CA-125. The physician has been monitoring therapy by following the trends in the CA-125 results. These patients' levels have been rising and were in the 90,000 U/mL range for their most recent result, but both results were now reported as "Too Big." The physician called the laboratory to determine what "Too Big" means. After calling up the results in the LIS, the laboratory director was able to report the first patient as 105,321 U/mL and the second patient as 125,090 U/mL. The director could not understand how the office received a "Too Big" result, since the numeric results were clearly displayed in the LIS. While the office was on the phone, the laboratory director logged into the clinical information system and reviewed these patients' results. In the electronic clinical information system, the results were both displayed as "Too Big." The director apologized for the issue and promised to contact information services to troubleshoot the problem.

Explanation and Consequences

Results can be altered during transmission between information systems. The laboratory is responsible for the accurate reporting and display of test results to the ordering physician. Initial interface verification of accurate result display should be periodically reverified for continued integrity of data transmission. Small changes in software and upgrades to the information system servers can affect interfaces and data transmission. In this case, the result interface could not handle results with 6 or more digits. Results of >100,000 U/mL are reported as "Too Big," meaning the result is too big for the computer interface to handle. Initial verification of this interface by the laboratory overlooked this anomaly, since all of the smaller results transmitted accurately. The problem was not discovered until a physician brought the result to the laboratory's attention. Electronic interfaces are complex, and verification of accurate data transmission and display should challenge the interface with more than routine results. Since high levels of analytes can occur, transmission at the extremes of the reportable range need to be confirmed as well, including results above and below the reportable range (with the < or > symbols). The laboratory should work with information services in the verification of electronic data interfaces in order to present cases that would challenge the verification process. Once connected, interfaces need ongoing monitoring to ensure ongoing quality.

> Information services can assist laboratory operations, particularly for the reporting of results to affiliated and nonaffiliated physician practices. While a goal of the EMR is to provide easy access to patient information as patients move throughout a health system (from inpatient to outpatient and to home health care), the stewards of the EMR also have the responsibility to protect the confidentiality of patient results and limit access to only those clinicians involved in the patient's care. The Health Insurance Portability and Accountability Act (HIPAA) of 1996 contains privacy regulations governing appropriate access to patient information. Determining and enforcing appropriate access to the EMR can be complicated, since patients may be seen at multiple sites, sometimes by physicians with competing clinical practices. Patients may seek advice from another physician in the form of a second opinion. Test results and medical record notes made by one physician should not necessarily be accessible to other physicians unless the results and records are released by the ordering physician or access is granted by the patient. Managing access can be complicated and presents a source for potential duplicative analysis and errors.

Case with Error

Two physicians are seeing the same patient and request identical chemistry and hematology tests. Although both physicians are affiliated with the health care system and laboratory performing the test, neither office has electronic records. In this case, the LIS prints test results and delivers the results via fax or hardcopy through the mail. Since both physicians ordered the same test, it would be more efficient for the laboratory to perform one analysis on one set of samples and print two copies for delivery of the results, one for each physician. However, the LIS can only generate one official result report per test request. All additional copies are reported as "Copy to Dr. . . ." The laboratory client service representatives wish to retain both physicians as clients, since they each send the laboratory a significant amount of business. One physician cannot receive an official report and the other a "copy to" report, since both are considered the primary ordering physician. Both must receive an official, original report. Since the LIS cannot handle two ordering physicians, two sets of samples must be collected from the patient and analyzed in order to generate two original result reports. This leads to more blood being collected from the patient and double the work for the laboratory without additional reimbursement, since the patient's insurance will only reimburse for one set of tests per day.

Explanation and Consequences

The LIS can facilitate laboratory efficiency or it can serve as an obstruction to efficient laboratory operations. In this case, the ability to only enter one ordering physician into the LIS record limited the ability of the system to send original result reports to more than one physician. A discussion of limitations needs to occur with information services to develop resolutions, or provide options for working around the limitations to best facilitate patient care and physician needs. While this case illustrated a problem providing hardcopy reports, similar limitations exist in EMR. One physician may not want access of results and notes on the patient written in his or her office to be available for other health care providers, especially if they are in competitive practices. Under HIPAA confidentiality regulations, laboratory results may only be released to the ordering physician or his or her delegates. Requests from other providers, even for the same test, may require separate analysis depending on the affiliations between organizations and office clients of the laboratory. As EMR and interfaces become more sophisticated, there may be new ways to resolve such conflicts in the future. Until then, laboratories will need to deal with conflicting requests and system limitations on a case-by-case basis.

STANDARDS OF CARE

▓ Test names can be confusing and laboratories must distinguish tests of similar names according to their clinical application, methodology, limitations, or other unique characteristics.

▓ Electronic ordering systems must facilitate physician ordering of the appropriate tests, while limiting the ability of physicians to bypass the system or continue to use written requisitions.

▓ Staff must check at least two unique patient identifiers with any patient interaction, particularly for patients with common or similar-sounding names, and staff should heed electronic system warnings that are intended to catch certain identification errors.

▓ Presentation of laboratory data for clinician review must be easily understood. Tests results can be displayed in tabular form in an EMR to show more results on a single screen and improve efficiency of review, but more data come with the risk of losing individual result comments or specimen details and the associated potential for clinical misinterpretation. Requiring staff to actively seek out specimen comments rather than passively displaying information with the result poses the risk that the staff will miss clinically significant details. Laboratories should use an information system that draws attention easily to important details, rather than making users work to find the information.

▓ While a goal of the EMR is to provide easy access to patient information as patients move throughout a health system (from inpatient to outpatient and home health care), stewards of the EMR must protect the confidentiality of patient results and limit access to only those clinicians involved in the patient's care.

▓ Laboratory staff must be involved in the verification process of electronic data interfaces, since they can pose real-life situations that will challenge the reliability of the interface. Once implemented, interfaces require ongoing monitoring to ensure consistent display of data, as minor changes and updates to an information system can lead to unintended interface issues.

7 Laboratory Safety

OVERVIEW

Safety is a key component of good laboratory practice and mandatory to permit basic operations to occur. Accidents occur because of unsafe workplace conditions. A first step to preventing accidents is to avoid unsafe conditions. The Occupational Safety and Health Administration (OSHA) is a federal agency concerned with employee safety and protection of employees from workplace injuries. OSHA enforces a number of federal regulations to ensure on-the-job safety for employees of all workplaces, not just the laboratory. A clinical laboratory presents particular hazards including exposure to patient specimens (with potential contact with infectious diseases and organisms, for example), chemicals, electrical risks from laboratory instruments, and needle exposures. An employee can be injured simply by moving heavy instrumentation or boxes of supplies. Phlebotomists can suffer puncture injury during specimen collection. Service representatives can be injured during analyzer maintenance and repair. Couriers driving specimens between physician offices and the laboratory can be hurt from accidents in vehicles and even slips or falls in icy and wet conditions. Specimen processors that utilize high-speed centrifuges to spin tubes and separate the cellular components of blood can present a danger of flying metal, tube breakage, and specimen aerosols when operated incorrectly or with equipment failure. Technologists can contact corrosive acids and bases, and be exposed to fumes from volatile solvents when preparing reagents. There are a significant number of potential safety hazards in a clinical laboratory.

Administration also needs to consider the potential for injury to others beyond their laboratory employees. Improper disposal of chemicals down drains and common sewer lines can contaminate water sources such as ponds, lakes, and drinking water reservoirs, and they can present other environmental hazards. Failure to clean portable laboratory analyzers between patients when testing at the point-of-care presents a risk of transmitting hepatitis, HIV, or noso-comial infections among patients. Thus, safe laboratory operations consider all sources and effects of potential harm to employees, patients, the general public, and the environment.

PREANALYTICAL ERRORS

Food Risks

▶ A first commandment of today's laboratory safety is pro-hibiting eating and drinking in the laboratory. When spec-imens are being processed, the opening and aliquoting of tubes and specimen containers present a risk of aerosols, spills, splashes, and other sources of contamination of food and drink. While this principle may now seem common sense to labora-tory technologists, managers, and directors, the hazards may not be so apparent when laboratory testing is actually conducted at the point-of-care by nurses.

Case with Error

A laboratory is conducting an inspection of nursing units to prepare for its inspection by an accreditation agency. The accreditation inspectors will be arriving unannounced, so the laboratory is preparing staff for the type of questions they will be asked and to look for any issues that would pose a potential citation during the inspection. While walking through the unit, the laboratory reviewer asks a nurse to confirm where point-of-care laboratory testing is conducted on the unit. The nurse points to an area of the counter behind the nursing station where there is a glucose meter, vial of urine dipsticks, control solutions, and a hemoglobin analyzer. On the counter, next to a sink is an open soda can. Coffee cups are drying on a rack behind the sink. Two cups of coffee and a plate of donuts are open on the counter and some staff are taking a break. When the laboratory reviewer shows concern over having drinks and food so close to where testing is occurring, the nurse says this should not be an issue since there is a line of tape on the counter. Laboratory testing only occurs on the right side of the tape, so staff can leave food and drinks on the counter as long as these are left on the left side of the tape.

Explanation and Consequences

Having food in close proximity to any location where patient blood and body fluids are being tested is an unsafe situation. The tape on the counter does not prevent a sample from splashing across the counter, or a specimen from spraying droplets when a stopper is removed from a tube. For this reason, specimen stoppers should be removed only behind a splash shield and staff should wear appropriate protective equipment, that is, gloves, lab coat, and safety glasses (or face mask if a protective shield is not available). This equipment protects staff from the potential exposure to blood or specimens during testing. While it may be acceptable to eat and drink at a nursing station while staff are discussing cases or reviewing medical records, laboratory testing should not take place in the same location. A utility room or soiled linen closet may be a better location for point-of-care testing (POCT) rather than a counter behind a high-traffic staff work area. Laboratory testing should be clearly separated from other functions involving food, medicines, or clean medical supplies on the nursing unit.

In addition, the close proximity of testing to a sink risks contaminating the laboratory reagents with water. Dipsticks, glucose test strips, and other POCT reagents are hygroscopic, and localizing testing close to a sink creates the potential for laboratory error from damp reagents. Storing urine dipsticks in a bathroom also risks exposure of those strips to water, changing their reactivity. Splashing of water onto the bottle label can further affect test results by discoloring the interpretation chart printed on every bottle. For a variety of reasons, laboratory testing should not occur at a busy nursing station close to food and water.

> Specimens that are spilled or splashed on countertops during testing can present a hazard if the countertops are not sufficiently cleaned after use. The presence of organisms (some of which may be resistant to antibiotics) risks a spread of nosocomial infections unless devices, reagents, and supplies are thoroughly cleaned and disinfected between patients. Contamination on countertops can be picked up on gloves and on the bottoms of reagent vials or meters and carried to other surfaces if adequate disinfection is not conducted after testing. Protective pads and other absorbent materials can help contain specimens, but may not completely prevent contact with surfaces underneath the pad. Eating and drinking using the same surface where testing is conducted present a risk to staff and others consuming the food.

Case with Error

A drug rehabilitation and residence facility conducts on-site urine drug and blood glucose testing on its patients. The drug testing is utilized to manage treatment and assess compliance during the program to ensure that patients are not continuing to abuse drugs during visits away from the facility. Blood glucose testing is available to manage insulin therapy for diabetic patients undergoing drug withdrawal. At this facility, space is limited, and the laboratory tests are thus conducted in the one examination room at the clinic. The remaining rooms are set up for group and individual counseling sessions. The laboratory at the local hospital assists with managing the test quality and staff education, training, and competency. During a monthly visit, laboratory staff note lunch being served on a counter in the examination room. The laboratory representative asks why food is set up in a patient examination room, and the clinical staff note that lunch is always set up in that room. Access to food can be controlled in the exam room, since the manager's office is directly opposite the examination room. Otherwise, the first people to arrive will consume all of the food before other staff and patients have an opportunity. The food, utensils, and drinks are observed to be on the same counter where the urine drug and blood glucose tests were just conducted. The nurse indicates that she wiped the counter with soap and water before setting up the sandwiches.

Explanation and Consequences

Safe laboratory operation requires delineation of clean and dirty areas of the laboratory. Phones, computers, and countertops that may be handled with gloved hands while manipulating specimens ("dirty" areas of the laboratory) are considered differently from phones, computers, and counters that are accessed without gloves and by visitors to the laboratory ("clean" areas of the laboratory). Potentially contaminated countertops and equipment should be regularly disinfected with a 1:10 dilution of bleach or other hospital-grade disinfectant to prevent spread of organisms by contact. However, bleach and other disinfectants are harsh and can also corrode plastics and surfaces. Cracks and crevices in the outer coating of equipment as well as countertop connections and grout can be difficult to clean and may continue to harbor blood, fluids, and organisms. Therefore, utilizing the same counters for laboratory testing and food service is a safety concern and should be avoided. Food service should be reserved for break rooms, office suites, and other locations physically and functionally separated from laboratory testing. Staff should be conscious of the potential for surface transmission of organisms, some of which may be resistant to antibiotics, take appropriate precautions when handling biologic specimens, and follow appropriate infection control policies.

> ▶ Consideration should be made for separation of clean linens, medications, and other supplies that could become contaminated in areas where laboratory testing is taking place. Food and medications that are intended for patient or employee consumption should not be stored in the same refrigerators as patient specimens or with potentially biohazardous controls or reagents made from blood products. Separate clean and dirty

refrigerators are recommended and should be clearly labeled as to their intended purpose. Likewise, food served in patient care areas requires consideration for separation of areas that are potentially infectious from clean areas.

Case with Error

A pharmaceutical vendor is providing lunch for participants in a continuing education activity in the emergency department (ED). Due to space constraints in the ED, the buffet lunch is set up outside the meeting room in the hallway next to the nursing admissions station. This is convenient as the nursing station is very busy, and staff can take food as they pass by, while they are admitting patients to rooms, and moving patients between rooms. Phlebotomy supplies and glucose meters are stored on the counter of the nursing station, and specimens that are ready to send to the laboratory by pneumatic tube are dropped off by staff on the same nursing station counter above the buffet table.

Explanation and Consequences

Placing food in an open hallway where patients are being transported is not a safe practice. Food service should be reserved for clean areas of a hospital, such as cafeterias and employee break rooms. Patient care areas where examinations and procedures are conducted have the potential to be contaminated with blood and body fluids. These areas are dirty, and should be managed as potentially contaminated, requiring periodic and regular disinfection between individual patients and certainly whenever visibly soiled. These are not appropriate areas for storing food or serving meals, no matter how busy the employees might be.

Chemical Hazards

▶ Safe laboratory operations require awareness of chemical hazards. Fumes from volatile chemicals can fill closed spaces and overwhelm staff. Such chemicals should be stored in vented cabinets and only utilized in fume hoods or rooms with adequate air exchange. Other chemicals can be hazardous when mixed, such as acids and bases. Metallic elements can become explosive in the presence of water. Laboratories need to carefully inventory the chemicals stored and utilized in their tests, provide for appropriate storage conditions, and ensure proper disposal.

Case with Error

A research laboratory involved with teaching and mentoring trainees in laboratory medicine has been involved in the development of several clinical assays over the years. During this time, the laboratory has amassed a large collection of chemicals and solvents utilized for specimen extraction and chromatography. Due to building renovations, the laboratory needs to temporarily relocate while new floors, ventilation systems, benches, and fume hoods are installed. Before the laboratory can move, the chemicals need to be assessed. All bottles have to be inventoried and old chemicals disposed of. During the inventory, the laboratory staff finds several cans of diethyl ether in the storage cabinet under the fume hood. The cans appear to be rusting, the labels are faded, and staff is not clear how old the cans may be or how to properly dispose of old ether. The laboratory contacts the chemical waste management department of the university who calls the local fire department and a bomb squad is sent to the laboratory for removal of the cans. The laboratory building had to be evacuated as well as an adjacent block surrounding the laboratory prior to chemical removal.

Explanation and Consequences

Diethyl ether is a highly flammable compound that can ignite on contact with flame or even warm surfaces. Peroxides can form as ether ages, forming diethyl ether peroxide that can explode on contact when dry. Storing ether in the laboratory requires consideration of its flammable potential and its risk of peroxide formation. Empty storage containers for all solvents must be promptly disposed of and expiration dates of laboratory stocks strictly monitored. Safe laboratory operations allow only certain quantities of ether to be stored in a single room without additional considerations for venting and fire hazard.

While this case made the evening news, ether is not the only chemical hazard found in a laboratory. Other chemicals present a risk of fire, fumes, burns, and other safety concerns for staff. For example, sodium azide, a chemical that once was commonly added as a bacteriocidal agent to increase the shelf life of laboratory reagents and buffers, presents a serious problem. Disposal of azide-containing reagents down a drain could allow the azide to react with lead in the pipes and create a highly explosive compound, lead azide, that is used in bomb detonators. Laboratories need to be aware of not only the chemicals that are stored in the laboratory, but also the components of prepackaged reagents utilized in their analyzers, and ensure proper storage and disposal of those compounds. As another example, older buildings have copper pipes with lead solder, so disposal of chemicals and used reagents down common drains in such buildings requires consideration of possible reactions with aged plumbing systems and ultimately the possibility for environmental contamination of waste water.

Transportation and Processing

Specimen storage and transport can also present hazardous situations. Couriers who transport specimens need to be concerned about the potential for container breakage and specimens leaking into cars or vans. The potential for a vehicle accident requires consideration that specimens could be released into the environment and contaminate surroundings. Specimens could be blood or body fluids containing agents for hepatitis or other bloodborne diseases, or, in a worst-case scenario, rare highly infectious pathogens destined for identification at state laboratories or the Centers for Disease Control and Prevention. This is why the Department of Transportation (DOT), the International Air Transport Association (IATA), and other agencies have enacted packaging and shipping regulations intended to contain specimens, even if they break in transit, to protect employees, the environment, and the general public from exposure during transit.

Case with Error

The processing center of a clinical laboratory manages a number of outpatient and inpatient specimens each day. These specimens come from regional physician offices by courier, as well as by shuttle from local phlebotomy stations. A fecal fat specimen was dropped off late in the afternoon from a physician's office for courier pickup. Fecal fat specimens are collected and transported in paint cans to prevent leakage of the specimen during transport. The office was closing early due to an upcoming holiday weekend, so the specimen was left in the drop box on the side of the building for pickup. As this was a 4th of July holiday weekend, specimen pickup occurred earlier that day, and this specimen missed the early pickup and sat in the heat over the weekend until the following Tuesday morning. By the time the specimen was delivered to the laboratory, the sides of the can were extended from increased pressure due to bacterial gas production. The paint can exploded in the specimen processing area of laboratory receiving, splattering the processing staff and the entire room with the patient's specimen. Fortunately, staff did not receive any cuts or serious injuries, but were directly exposed to the patient's stool specimen. The processing center had to be closed and sandblasted prior to painting before the room could be used again.

Explanation and Consequences

Heating a closed system can have explosive consequences. Fecal fat specimens are now collected and transported in vented containers to prevent buildup of gas within the container. Additional safety precautions when opening specimen containers in a fume hood should be enacted to both contain any specimen spilled during opening and limit exposure of the person processing the specimen should the specimen explode. Safety policies need to consider the possibility of specimen breakage, leaks, and even explosions during transportation and processing. Transportation packaging should contain the specimen if it is released from the tube, and limit exposure of the specimen contents to the environment. Double packaging with absorbent material and waterproof bags provide a cushion for the specimen from breakage, but also contain the specimen if the sample does leak. Additional precautions are also necessary for certain pathogens or suspected diseases to provide extra levels of containment if the specimen leaks in transit.

> ▶ Laboratory instrumentation can present a safety hazard. Automated analyzers have a number of moving parts, and performing repairs and maintenance on working analyzers can lead to operator injury. Staff can be cut or punctured by moving probes, suffer electrical shock if they come into contact with the instrument after water leaks into the circuitry of the instrument, and be exposed to chemicals and body fluids if protective covers are moved during operation. Every area of the laboratory presents a safety risk if policies and procedures are not implemented to alert employees to the potential for harm. Staff should never run equipment without sufficient training, and should always take precautions to ensure appropriate operation whenever working with laboratory equipment.

Case with Error

The processing staff in a clinical laboratory were preparing samples for analysis. Tubes of blood were loaded manually into the carriers of a centrifuge and spun for several minutes to separate cells from serum for testing. The centrifuges have been well maintained, and the speed recently calibrated. However, a number of specimen tubes were noted to be breaking during centrifugation (a few tubes each week). Each time this occurred, the centrifuge was out of operation for over an hour for cleaning and disinfection. During one run, a tube broke during centrifugation and the centrifuge lid lifted sufficiently to allow shards of plastic to fly out of the centrifuge across the laboratory. Although no one was injured, the plastic did ricochet off countertops, floors, and walls, imbedding into an office divider across the room before the centrifuge could be stopped. In the interim, staff were ducking under benches and running for cover to avoid being hit with debris.

Explanation and Consequences

While the centrifuge was well maintained, specimens were being spun without a cover on the rotor baskets. The basket covers contain any fluids that may leak from the specimens during centrifugation, and allow for easier cleanup of spills, since only the tube carriers need to be cleaned rather than the entire interior of the centrifuge. The basket covers also provide a smooth surface to reduce friction from air flow during centrifugation. Spinning tubes at high speeds without the basket cover forces air flow around and between the tubes, producing turbulence during the run. The added shear forces contributed to the increased frequency of tube breakage in the centrifuge.

The latch also did not function properly on this centrifuge. The latch should lock the entire centrifuge lid in place during operation. This failed locking mechanism allowed the lid to rise during operation, allowing an opening for tube fragments and liquid specimen to exit the centrifuge. The rotor is spinning the tubes at such high speed that any remnant of broken tubes will be exiting at high speed, with a force that could possibly cause grave injury to any staff in the near vicinity. A correctly functioning latch should allow the lid to seal the centrifuge during operation and contain any specimen leaks or breakage.

Staff should have read the owner's manual for the centrifuge and received instruction from the manufacturer prior to use. The owner's manual clearly indicates that the centrifuge should never be operated without covers on the specimen baskets. The added turbulence from improper operation may have contributed to specimen breakage and could also have caused the latch to not seal completely during operation.

STANDARDS OF CARE

■ Staff should be cognizant of infection-control policies, the potential for surface contamination, and the need for routine cleaning and disinfection.
■ DOT and IATA safety and shipping regulations must be enforced to protect employees handling specimens, the environment, and the general public from exposure to biohazardous pathogens.

- Personal protective equipment, that is, gloves, lab coat, safety glasses, and splash shields, must be used appropriately to protect staff from potential exposure to blood or fluids during specimen manipulation.
- There must be separation of clean supplies, such as linens, medications, and medical equipment, from areas where laboratory testing is taking place.
- Surfaces, such as countertops, medical equipment, testing devices, beds, railings, and nightstands, can become contaminated with antibiotic-resistant organisms and require regular cleaning and disinfection, especially when shared between patients.
- Chemicals that present a risk of fire, fumes, burns, or other safety concerns for staff require handling, storage, and disposal according to specific guidelines.
- Staff should never run equipment without training and should always take precautions to ensure appropriate operation whenever working with laboratory equipment.

RECOMMENDED READING

International Air Transport Association. *Dangerous goods regulations manual*. 54th ed. Geneva, Switzerland: International Air Transport Association; 2013.

U.S. Pipeline and Hazardous Materials Safety Administration, Department of Transportation. Code of federal regulations, subchapter C, hazardous materials regulations. CFR 49, Part 171–173. October 1, 2011.

Outreach Testing

OVERVIEW

Outreach testing is an extension of a hospital laboratory to test samples from outside the institution, such as the region around the laboratory, including from private physician office practices, other hospitals, long-term care facilities, and other sites. Increasing the outpatient volume of samples increases laboratory profitability, since insurance companies currently pay for laboratory tests as a fee for service on a per-test basis for outpatient visits. In contrast, there is a single flat reimbursement for inpatients for all costs incurred based on a diagnosis that encompasses the entire treatment. Thus, many hospitals are seeking to expand their laboratory testing market by partnering with local physician offices. Outreach testing programs are a growing business model as health care finances get tighter.

The outreach business model provides advantages for both parties. Physicians will have access to local expertise in the laboratory, while the hospital receives the additional sample volume. Physician offices find local laboratories more accessible, and on that basis, more responsive to inquiries, as compared with national reference laboratories that may have automated answering machines and may require multiple transfers to reach someone who is knowledgeable enough to manage their question.

Unfortunately, an outreach business based on profit and client growth can sometimes be at odds with inpatient cost containment and test utilization strategies. Hospital laboratories engaging in outreach will need to invest in a sales and marketing staff, which was not a consideration prior to outreach. At least some of the sales staff may have never worked in a laboratory and may not realize the medical applications of specific tests or method limitations and interferences. Their job is to satisfy clients and provide better service than the national reference laboratories against whom they are competing. While medical directors may be ensuring that inpatient physicians order the right test for a specific patient's suspected condition and limit test overutilization, outreach sales personnel are promoting physician ordering and inadvertently, or otherwise, overordering. For outreach work, there is emphasis on the old business adage that the client is always right. While medical directors may seek to limit or place an "approval-only ordering" rule on certain high-cost esoteric tests, for inpatients, the goal of outreach sales is to facilitate their clients' ability to get any test to keep the account. Conflicts can arise when physicians can freely order esoteric and routine tests for their office patients, but are limited and restricted from ordering the same tests on their inpatients. This dynamic creates the potential for laboratory miscommunication, conflict, and errors. While standardization across the system may be best, budgets and politics may limit a laboratory's ability to implement one-size-fits-all policies across all inpatient, outpatient, and outreach operations.

PREANALYTICAL ERRORS

▶ Common policies and procedures should be the goal throughout an organization. However, outreach programs are often managed by business managers, while inpatient laboratory operations are more directly supervised by medical directors. This creates two separate business operations within the laboratory, sometimes with different and conflicting goals and policies. Problems can occur when communication breaks down between the two operations, and the outreach managers develop policies and procedures independent of existing laboratory operations.

Case with Error

The outreach program for a hospital system maintains a stock of supplies for physician office clients. These supplies are audited and documented for each physician office. Federal compliance regulations mandate that laboratories cannot provide business incentives to their clients such as free tubes, gloves, and other disposables. Because of this, outreach programs must monitor the amount of supplies delivered to the client compared to the number of specimens received to ensure balance and compliance with federal regulations. In this hospital system, the outreach supplies are stored in a separate warehouse from the hospital products. This warehouse is at ambient temperature and can become quite warm in the summer (>110°F) and cold in the winter (<10°F). This was not considered a concern by the outreach managers, since the supplies are plastic disposable containers and collection equipment: needles, syringes, tourniquets, gauze, and disinfectants.

In the first year after expanding their outreach program, the hospital laboratory started experiencing a number of problems with their automated chemistry systems. The probes were becoming coated with gel, and gel was getting stuck in the pipettes. Inspection of the specimen tubes demonstrated a firm separation of cells from plasma/ serum, but the plasma portion of the specimen had a coating of gel floating on top of some of the specimens. This floating gel was clogging the pipettors and attaching to the sample probes. Upon further investigation, the specimens with these problems were coming from the outreach clients. The laboratory suspected that the centrifuges in outreach processing may be causing the incomplete specimen separation. However, to further investigate the problem, the laboratory also requested some of the outreach tubes from storage as part of the investigation. The collection tubes had an odd appearance. Gel separator tubes normally have a pellet of gel at the bottom of the tube prior to use. The outreach tubes had gel on the sides of the tubes and also into the stoppers. Apparently the gel in the tubes was melting during storage and was flowing inside the tube depending on the angle the tube was stored. The centrifuge maintenance records indicated that these instruments had been well maintained and functioning appropriately. The gel in the collection tubes was the culprit, and overheating of tubes in the warehouse seemed to be separating the components of the gel. Once melted, the gel did not reconstitute during specimen collection and processing. Some of the gel remained a solid and provided cell separation, but the rest of the gel remained liquid and floated above the sample, affecting specimen analysis. The compromised stock was destroyed and new storage was arranged in a temperature-controlled warehouse. No further issues with gel on the analyzer probes were noted.

Explanation and Consequences

Storage conditions for reagents and supplies are a laboratory function, and sales staff may not be aware of the need for controlled conditions or the consequences from exposure of supplies to temperature extremes. By setting up two separate supplies, the hospital met federal compliance regulations, but medical director oversight was also overlooked in this case. The outreach program developed specimen storage conditions separate from current laboratory policy, without medical director review and agreement. Placing the supplies under different management structures shifted responsibilities for the outreach supplies and shifted oversight of the technical components of the supply storage. Outreach programs should ensure continuity of clinical oversight as they develop, as well as general and technical supervision, as required by U.S. federal CLIA regulations. While administration may consider CLIA to only apply to the analytical phase of laboratory testing, the overall quality of the test result is dependent on all phases of the testing process: preanalytical, analytical, and postanalytical. Outreach programs should ensure appropriate provision of medical and technical input into program operations.

> Medical director participation in the management of hospital outreach programs is required to adequately recognize and prevent certain errors. Medical directors have a perspective on the clinical utilization of test results as well as preanalytical sources of error that sales and administrative staff in hospital outreach programs may not appreciate. What may seem to be a minor change in practice could lead to significant effects on patient results. Operational changes should be routinely reviewed by a medical director for potential issues.

Case with Error

The outreach manager of the laboratory is approached by a laboratory supply vendor. This company can offer blood collection tubes with a savings of 0.1 cents per tube. Over the course of a year, this could save the hospital $50,000–$60,000. The outreach manager signs a contract with the purchasing department, and begins replacing the current tube supply over the next month.

Shortly after the change is made, the analyzing laboratory begins to notice specimens are being received in a different type of tube. Upon inquiry, the laboratory discovers that it is actually department staff from the outreach section that signed off on the change in tubes. No validation was performed on the tubes, and the laboratory is not certain of the impact of changing collection tubes. The new collection tube is constructed of a different type of plastic, and the gel separator is proprietary to this company. The gel could bind drugs and proteins differently than the current tubes. The length of storage and contact of a specimen with the gel could be a concern. Additionally, chemicals used in hardening the plastic of the tube and rubber stoppers could leach into the sample over time, potentially interfering with some colorimetric tests, immunoassays, and chromatographic assays. Short of thoroughly evaluating the new collection tube, the test results for specimens that were already reported include a warning to "interpret results with caution." The director also engages the purchasing department to suspend release of additional collection tubes from the new vendor until the laboratory can thoroughly compare results between the new and current collection tubes for all analytes tested in the laboratory.

Explanation and Consequences

Engaging staff and directors with technical knowledge and experience with changes to laboratory operations is a critical component of good laboratory management. Although one section of laboratory administration could see a financial benefit from switching collection tubes, this staff did not recognize the full ramifications of implementing a new tube. The cost of validating a new collection tube would exceed any potential financial savings expected from adopting the tube, and should have been part of the decision to change tube manufacturers. Some hospitals have New Technology Committees to facilitate the review and implementation of new and revised products. A New Technology Committee is tasked with evaluating the benefits and risks of converting to new technology. Many departments should be involved in the decision-making process. A committee format ensures that everyone has an opportunity to review the product and offer an opinion. Had this case gone through a committee process, the laboratory director would likely have had the opportunity to discuss the potential consequences of changing tubes, and describe the necessary evaluations that must be performed before implementation. Contracts could have been drafted as contingent on successful performance of the tube in these evaluations. Those involved with the current case did not appreciate the need for evaluation, much less a problem arising during the evaluation. Nursing units and phlebotomy practice could also be affected if the new collection tube requires special adapters or additional disposables associated with blood collection. Thus, a New Technology Committee is one way to provide opportunity for staff with a stake in a product to offer an opinion for the entire committee to consider.

A laboratory is sometimes the consumer rather than the provider of laboratory testing. No single laboratory can perform all possible tests that could be ordered by hospital staff or physician offices. At one time or another, every laboratory must send a sample to another laboratory for analysis. This may occur because the volume of a particular test is low, the test requires specialized equipment or staffing, or the test is so esoteric that the laboratory simply cannot set up the test. Certain tests are also proprietary and are only performed by one laboratory. As a consumer of laboratory tests, clinical staff can get a different impression of customer service offered by a laboratory because the test requested is actually performed by a different laboratory. Difficulties reaching someone who can answer a question or inconsistencies in results between outside laboratories can leave the physician with a poor impression of laboratory quality.

Case with Error

A hospital laboratory with a moderate-size outreach program utilizes a national reference laboratory for analysis of lead specimens. The reference laboratory offers testing at a cost that is lower than the hospital laboratory can provide internally. So, the hospital laboratory sends all lead requests to the national reference laboratory for analysis, and the pediatricians associated with the hospital have been pleased with the service.

The reference laboratory is composed of a network of several regional laboratories and a central headquarters analyzing facility. While lead testing from this hospital had been performed for many years at one of the regional laboratories, as the number of requests grew, the reference laboratory started sending specimens to its central headquarters for analysis. Within the first week of sample testing at the reference laboratory headquarters, the hospital began to receive complaints from its pediatricians about the number of results reported with the comment: "quantity not sufficient for analysis." More than half the 50 specimens analyzed in the first week of analysis were clotted or had an insufficient quantity of specimen to complete the analysis.

When the hospital complained to the reference laboratory, it took several calls and messages to reach a technical supervisor in person.

After discussing the problem, the supervisor could only state that the laboratory has always had a policy to comment that specimens could be compromised and that the hospital utilize the correct specimen container. Apparently, the regional laboratory had no collection container recommendations, while the headquarters laboratory had specific recommendations for a particular manufacturer and type of microtainer tube. When the hospital called the regional laboratory, no checks on specimen quality were performed prior to analysis, and results were never associated with a qualifying statement unless there was not enough specimen volume for analysis. The regional laboratory required half the specimen volume of the headquarters laboratory. When the hospital pointed out the inconsistencies in practice between two sites owned and operated under the same reference laboratory name, the local sales representative just shrugged and asked if the hospital would rather have their specimens sent back to the regional laboratory.

Explanation and Consequences

Inconsistencies are a sign of poor service and quality. Inconsistencies in test results or laboratory response to an issue make the client question the quality of the laboratory. When a system has multiple locations for analysis of an analyte, the laboratory has an obligation to correlate the results between analyzing locations. CLIA requires correlation between different analyzers within the same location and under the same license. However, when laboratories have multiple testing locations under different licenses, the organization needs to think more globally about consistency in methods, performance, and results. The result carries the corporate name regardless of where the test was analyzed within an organization. When one location recommends different collection tubes and utilizes different processing procedures, questions arise regarding the potential for disagreement of test results between the different laboratory facilities. In this case, the response by the reference laboratory is paramount to maintaining the client's faith in the laboratory. Unfortunately, the response was inconsistent and inadequate in this case. When concordance of results between multiple analytical sites may not be possible, the laboratory must clearly define for its users the nature of the differences and what those differences mean for clinical interpretation of the test results.

POSTANALYTICAL ERRORS

▶The complexity of multiple laboratories performing and billing for specimen analysis can be confusing to physicians and patients. The laboratory performing a test is generally responsible for billing the patient's insurance. If the insurance company does not cover the costs of the test or only partially reimburses, then the patient may be responsible for the difference. Therefore, the patient may receive a bill from both the physician's office for a visit, and a separate bill from the laboratory for tests associated with that visit. When a hospital laboratory cannot perform the requested test and the specimen is sent to a referral laboratory, the hospital laboratory may receive the bill from the referral laboratory directly. The hospital laboratory is then responsible for billing and recovering the referral laboratory charges from either the patient's insurance or the patient directly. If neither pays, then the hospital laboratory suffers the loss. Some reference laboratories, however, will directly bill the patient's insurance ("third-party billing") and will take on the financial risk if the insurance or patient does not pay. In such cases, patients may receive a bill for test results from an unfamiliar laboratory.

Case with Error

A patient calls the family physician that she has been seeing for years. The patient has been having periodic bouts with diarrhea despite changes in diet to try to relieve the diarrhea. The physician on the last visit recommends a new test for inflammatory bowel disease. The blood tests are collected in the physician's office and picked up by a courier from the hospital laboratory across the street. All testing from this physician's office is usually performed by the hospital laboratory.

The patient was calling to complain about a bill for several hundred dollars they received from a GI specialty laboratory. The patient did not recognize this laboratory, and never had blood collected by this laboratory. The bill was for testing that the patient could not pronounce, but indicated that the patient's insurance company denied the claim so the patient was responsible for the cost of the test. The physician does not understand the problem and calls the hospital laboratory. The hospital does not perform the test requested by the physician, so the specimens were forwarded by the hospital to an outside GI specialty laboratory for analysis.

Explanation and Consequences

Referral laboratory testing and billing can be complicated. The costs of laboratory tests, insurance reimbursement rates, and out-of-pocket expense to the patient are impacted by the site of care and are not predictable for physicians and patients. Ordering physicians have the responsibility to discuss the benefits and limitations of diagnostic testing. Part of that discussion should involve the clinical advantages, disadvantages, and financial consequences of performing the test. This information allows patients to make an informed decision about the value of the test to their management and whether they are prepared for the costs. Physicians should also discuss whether the patient will be receiving a bill from the physician's office, the hospital laboratory, or some other laboratory, so that the patient can be prepared when receiving unfamiliar mail. Most tests require the physician to document medical necessity for the tests to be reimbursed by an insurance company. For some esoteric tests, prior authorization may also be required by the patient's insurance company to cover the costs of the test. Laboratories may need the patient to sign an Advanced Beneficiary Notice (ABN) to indicate that the patient may be responsible for the cost of the test if the patient's insurance provider does not pay for the test. The laboratory should partner with physicians to ensure that they are up-to-date with current testing trends, costs, reimbursement trends, and the menu of tests performed internally versus those tests referred to other laboratories.

Laboratories have the responsibility for timely reporting of test results to outreach clients, just as they would for their own hospitalized inpatients. Unfortunately, many outreach clients are physician offices that are closed after hours. These offices may have intermittent coverage that can present a challenge to laboratories that need to reach the ordering physician after hours.

Case with Error

A hospital outreach program is acquiring a new physician practice as a client. The physician office does not have an after-hours answering service and has requested that the laboratory leave any critical results on the answering machine to be picked up during the next business day. As this is a client request, the sales staff approaches the laboratory director indicating that they must leave any critical-result communication on this physician's answering machine and not to bother him after hours.

Explanation and Consequences

A critical result is a laboratory value that represents a life-threatening clinical situation and requires immediate communication to a physician. Laboratories are required by federal CLIA law to contact the ordering physician or a designated staff member who can take clinical action to report a critical result. The laboratory must contact a live person to communicate a critical result as soon as possible and verify read-back understanding of the communication. Laboratories cannot leave a message for a physician to pick up at a later time. An office answering service can be contacted if it results in a call to the physician, or the physician can be paged to indicate that the laboratory has a critical value on one of the clinic's patients. The physician or designee must physically return the laboratory's call to verbally acknowledge receipt of the value and read back the result to confirm correct understanding. Therefore, in this case, the laboratory cannot legally comply with the sales staff request and must have a means of contacting someone who is responsible for patient care after hours, typically the ordering physician or a covering physician/clinical staff member.

STANDARDS OF CARE

▓ Laboratory outreach expands the current laboratory operations beyond the walls of the hospital, but uniform policies and procedures must be in place to ensure comparable quality of testing.

▓ A New Technology Committee provides a forum for stakeholders to review the advantages, limitations, and financial consequences of using a new product or laboratory test. Such a committee should be implemented to develop consensus decisions for new technology, including laboratory testing.

▓ Ordering physicians have the responsibility to discuss the benefits and limitations of diagnostic testing with patients.

▓ A laboratory must inform physicians to make them up-to-date with current testing trends, costs, and the menu of tests performed internally as well as the tests referred to other laboratories.

▓ A critical result is a laboratory value that represents an imminently life-threatening clinical situation and requires immediate communication to a physician. The laboratory must contact a clinician in real time, either the ordering physician or their designee who can take clinical action, to communicate a critical result and verify accurate understanding of the communication via read-back. Hospital outreach is a business model for expanding laboratory services that require sales and marketing administration, but clinical and technical oversight of the operation also requires medical director participation.

▓ Hospital outreach that facilitates any test that a physician wants may sometimes be at odds with hospital laboratory goals of limiting test utilization. Communication is essential between outreach sales staff who may have little laboratory experience and the laboratory staff and medical directors with extensive clinical and technical experience.

Index